EAT YOURSELF SMARTER!

The Ultimate Brain-Food Diet

MICHELLE STACEY

CENTENNIAL BOOKS

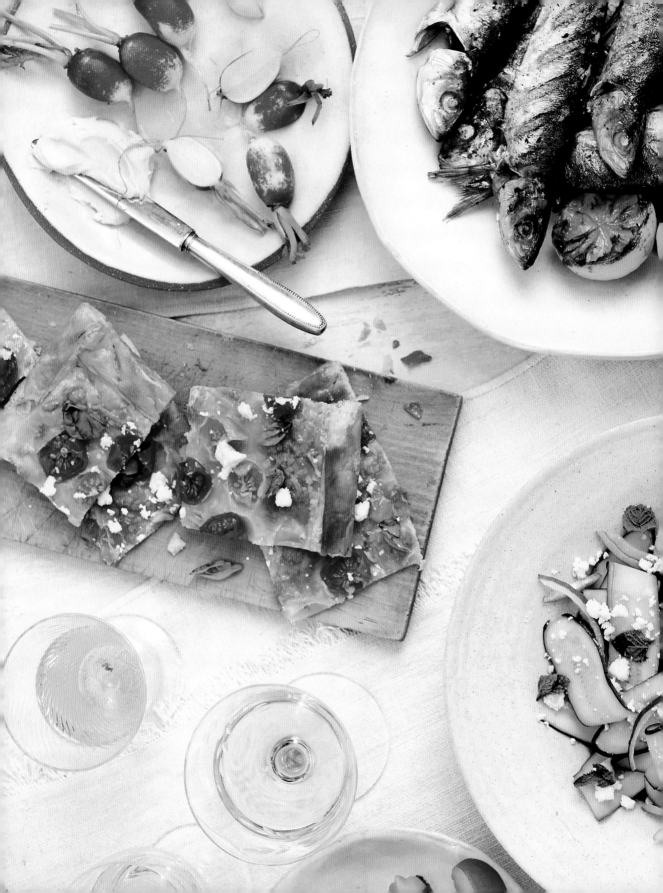

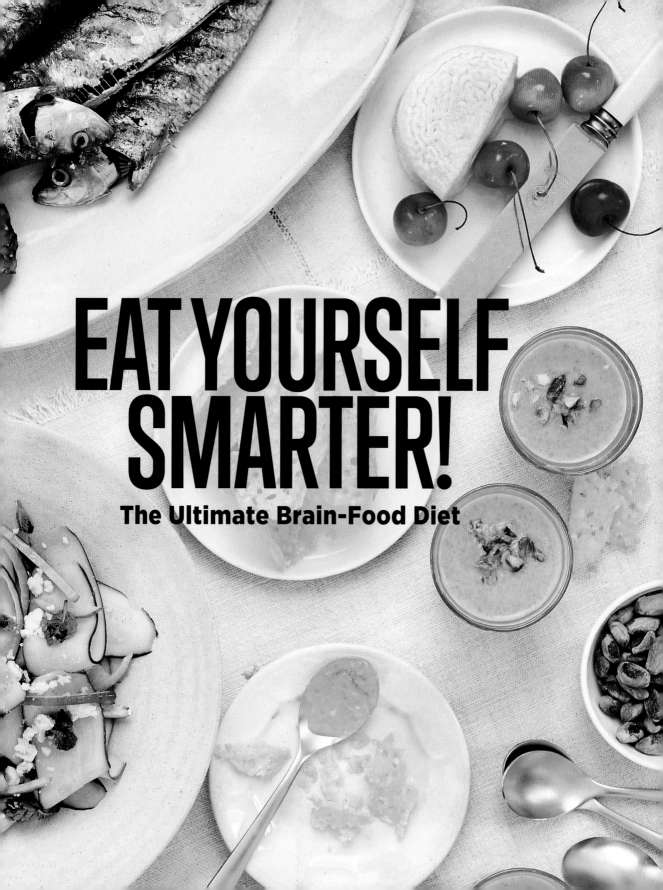

EAT YOURSELF SMARTER!

The Ultimate Brain-Food Diet

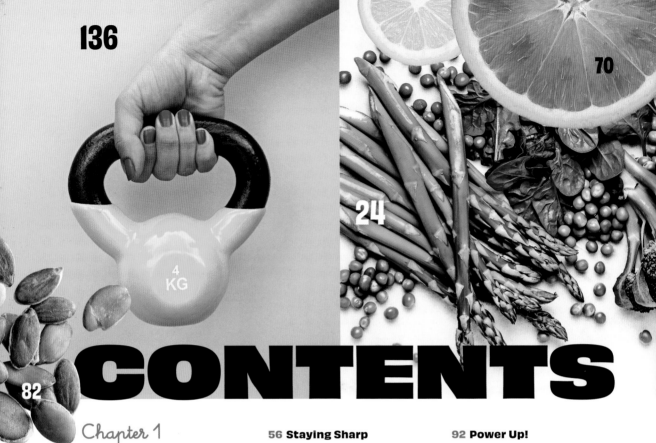

136

70

24

82

CONTENTS

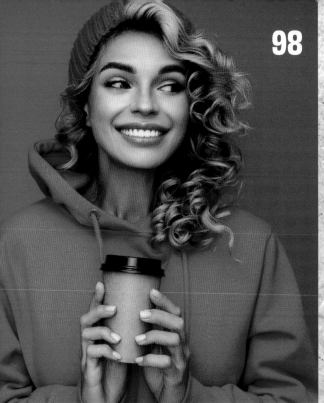

98

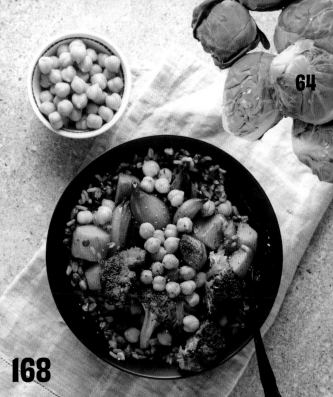

64

168

Chapter 4
GENIUS RECIPES

92

Feed Your Brain

* **YOUR DIETARY CHOICES CAN MAKE A BIG DIFFERENCE IN HOW YOU THINK AND FEEL.**

Good food equals good health. This basic concept has long been a no-brainer—baby boomers were raised on Wonder Bread's iconic tagline, "Helps Build Strong Bodies 12 Ways!" And despite the fact that packaged white bread has had a precipitous fall from grace since the 1960s, it's even more of a given these days that the right nutrition can fortify your heart, muscles, bones and teeth, while boosting energy and strength. But it's only recently that science has acknowledged the powerful effect that certain foods have on the health of arguably the body's most important organ of all: the brain.

Reams of research, plus sophisticated tools like functional MRIs, show that what you eat has a profound effect on how your brain operates. From cognitive function to better memory to happier moods, the nutrients you take in can shape your experience of the world, and it's all due to how nutrients affect the neurons and synapses in the brain.

In short, the path to a nimble, more resilient brain leads directly to the kitchen, and this book serves as a guide along that path. It can be as simple as loading up on the planet's smartest foods, which directly spur neurogenesis and neuroplasticity (the processes that create new brain cells and rewire them to work more efficiently), while avoiding those that slow or gum up that growth. And you'll learn how specific nutrients impact inflammation and the microbiome—which are key to cognitive function.

Get ready to say goodbye to brain fog and bad moods, and hello to a brighter, calmer, more focused new you.

— *Michelle Stacey*

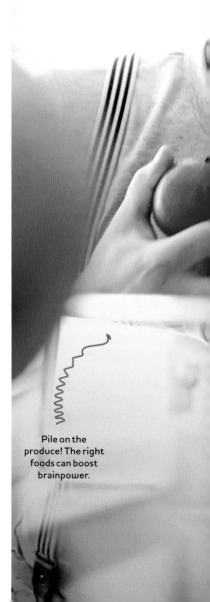

Pile on the produce! The right foods can boost brainpower.

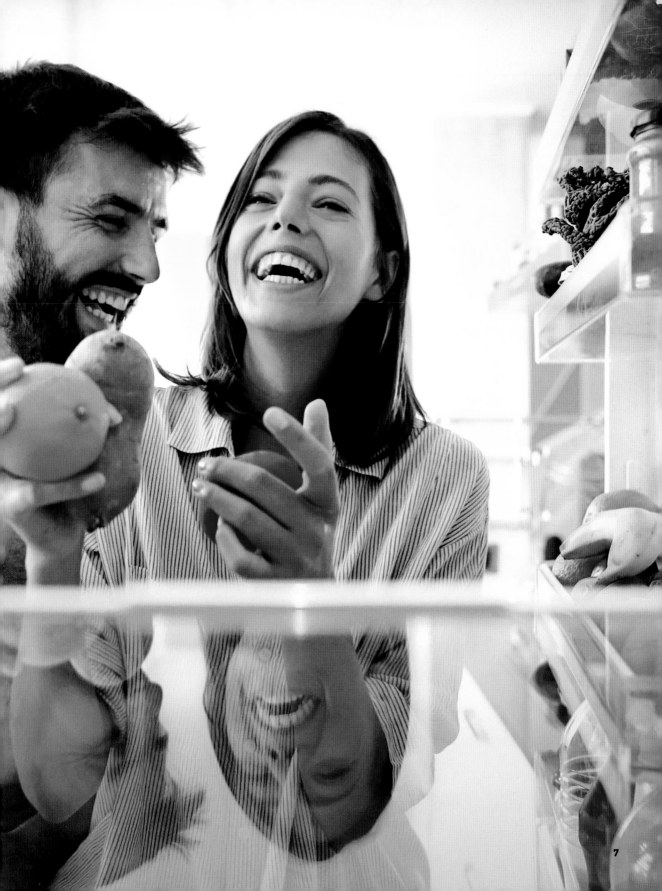

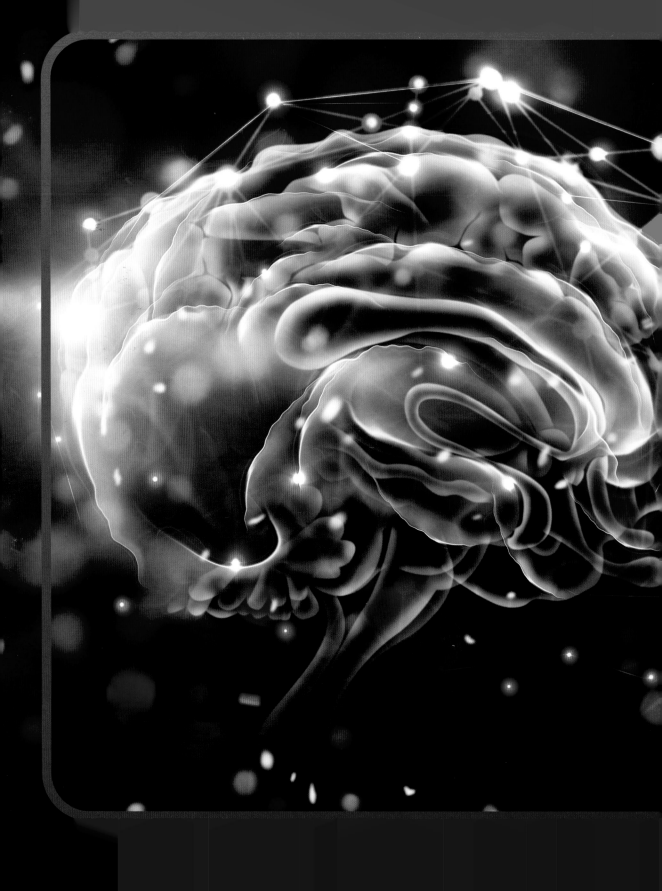

CHAPTER I

The Science of

SMART

WHAT WE'VE LEARNED—SO FAR—ABOUT
THE POWER OF NUTRITION TO BOOST
BRAIN FUNCTION AND IMPEDE AGING.

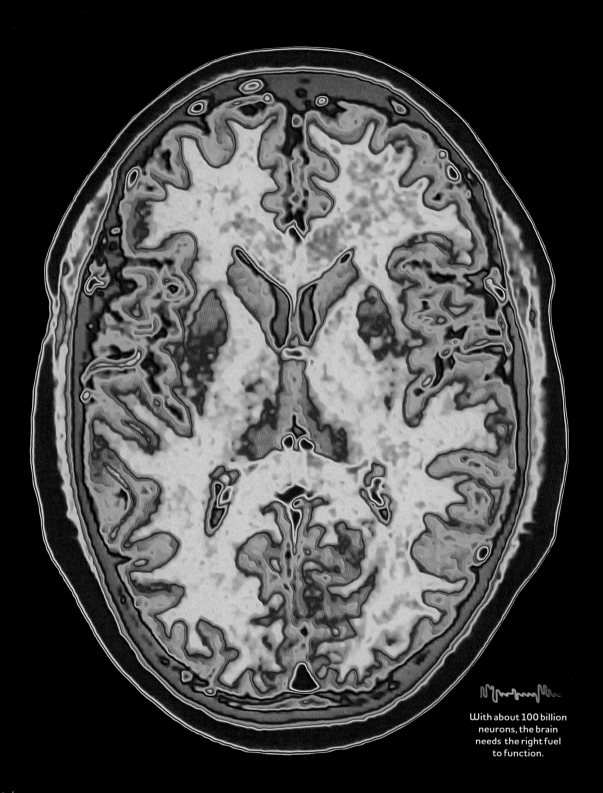

With about 100 billion neurons, the brain needs the right fuel to function.

The
BRAIN-FOOD REVOLUTION

* "YOU ARE WHAT YOU EAT" NOW HAS A WHOLE NEW MEANING, AS SCIENCE CATCHES UP TO THE IDEA THAT THE RIGHT FOODS FUEL NOT JUST YOUR MUSCLES BUT, CRUCIALLY, YOUR MOST IMPORTANT ORGAN: YOUR BRAIN.

For most of human history, we have thought of food as, essentially, fuel. We know we can't survive without it, that our organs, tissues and muscles need sustenance on a regular basis to continue to function. More recently, researchers have delved into that sustenance on a more specific, even molecular level: Which foods make us stronger? Healthier? More long-lived? We have learned vast amounts in just the past few decades about what constitutes "health food," and also which foods might be damaging to our bodies. Now we know, for instance, that a diet high in fresh fruits and vegetables may help protect against heart disease and cancer,

and that eating too many carbs and sweets can increase the risk of type 2 diabetes.

Amid all this knowledge, though, scientists are playing catch-up when it comes to food's effect on the function of one organ in particular—and ironically, it is the "hungriest" organ of all. The average human brain comprises only 2% of the body's weight, but it gobbles up about 20% of the calories we take in. It also doesn't thrive on just any old calories, according to neuroscientist Lisa Mosconi, PhD, associate director of the Alzheimer's Prevention Clinic at Weill Cornell Medical College/ New York-Presbyterian Hospital and author of *Brain Food: The Surprising Science of Eating*

for Cognitive Power. Instead, it is a spectacularly "picky eater," Mosconi notes. Certain nutrients have been key to humans becoming the high-functioning mammals we are today. "Our brain health is highly dependent on the food choices we make," says Mosconi. And increasingly, as our food supply has become more industrialized and further from what nature intended, we've been making some bad choices, brain-wise.

SCIENTIFIC WAKE-UP CALL

The intricate relationship between the foods we eat and the way we think and feel was, rather astonishingly, given little attention until recently. "When I

As we stray from home-cooked, whole foods (our brains' favorites), we suffer more from diseases of aging—including dementia.

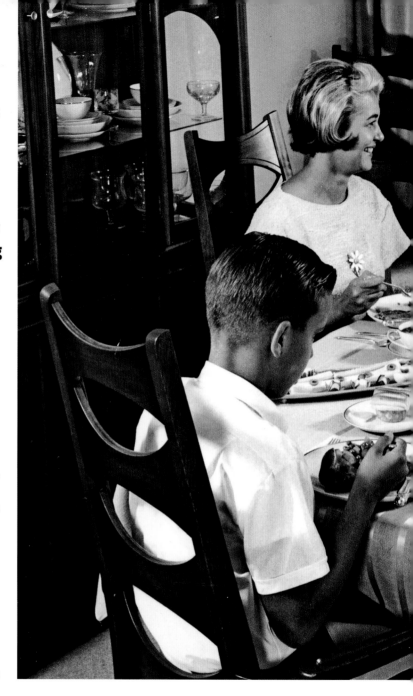

was studying neuroscience at Yale Medical School in the late 1970s, there wasn't a single nutrition course in the entire curriculum," says Louann Brizendine, MD, a neuropsychiatrist and author of *The Female Brain* and *The Male Brain.* "It just wasn't considered that important. And even now, only 25% of medical schools have nutrition courses." Medicine was, and in many ways continues to be, more focused on finding drug therapeutics to promote brain health—say, by seeking an "anti-Alzheimer's" medication— than on finding out how the food we give our brains, day in and day out, could influence the way that all-important organ works.

Even the scientists themselves seem taken aback by how key nutrition can be to brain function. As recently as 2015, a study in the journal *Foods* looking at the role of nutrients called xanthophylls—a type of carotenoid found in fruits and vegetables such as papaya, squash, peppers and leafy greens—found that these nutrients have a "multitude of functions" within the brain. "This field of study is relatively new, despite knowing that carotenoids could be found, even within the brain itself, for nearly 40 years," the researchers wrote. "It is perhaps surprising that it has taken us this long to study how foods, and the components of which they are composed, influence critically important

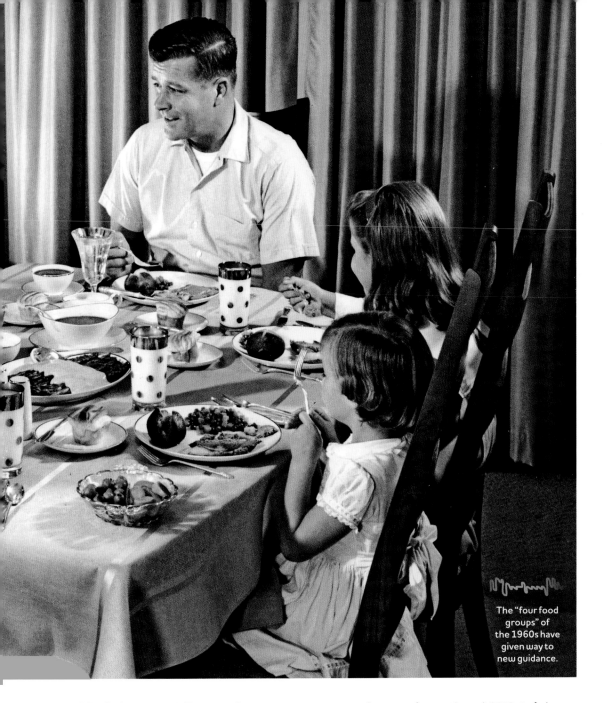

The "four food groups" of the 1960s have given way to new guidance.

tissues like the brain. Disciplines such as psychology and nutrition have rarely interacted in the past. This appears to be changing."

That change has been brought about, in part, by advances in imaging. Through MRIs and other scans, we can now see how various diets can change the very structure of our brains, rather than simply guessing based on more opaque methods like memory tests or, as our ancestors did, from subjective behavioral observations. A 2018 study in the journal *Neurology* followed almost 4,500 participants for 10 years, tracking their diets and giving them periodic brain MRIs. The researchers found that "better diet quality"—which

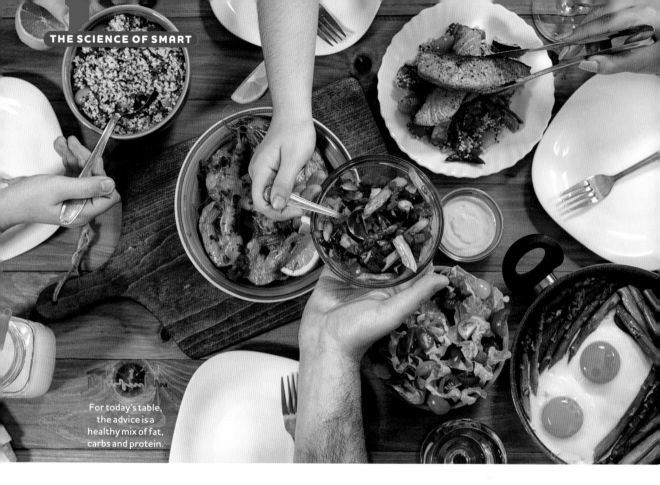

For today's table, the advice is a healthy mix of fat, carbs and protein.

they described as "high intake of vegetables, fruit, whole grains, nuts, dairy and fish, and low intake of sugar-containing beverages"—was associated with larger brain volumes. Many other studies have shown similar results; and when it comes to your brain, bigger *is* better.

Mosconi describes looking at scans comparing the brains of two middle-aged women: one who has been on a Mediterranean-type diet most of her life (similar to the diet tested in the *Neurology* study) and one who has been eating a Western-style diet for many years, meaning fast foods, processed meats, refined sweets and sodas and lower amounts of fresh fruits and vegetables. The Mediterranean-diet woman's brain looked healthy, says Mosconi—her brain took up most of the space inside the skull, and the hippocampus appeared well rounded and in contact with surrounding tissues.

In comparison, the brain of the Western-diet woman "showed brain atrophy, or shrinkage, an indicator of neuronal loss." Neurons are the basic working unit of the brain; they're specialized cells designed to transmit information to other nerve, muscle or gland cells. The hippocampus and temporal lobe in the Western-diet woman's brain, both regions directly involved in memory formation, were smaller and surrounded by fluid. "These are all signs of accelerated aging and increased risk of future dementia," Mosconi says. So yes, your brain health *is* influenced by what you eat.

IN THE BEGINNING

On the most basic level, a better diet is what allowed our species to become "human" at all—which in turn dictates why our brains are so demanding of certain nutrients. From prehistoric times to the present, our brains have more than tripled in size, says Mosconi, "largely thanks to changes in our ancestors' diets and eating habits." For millions of years, our precursors' brains were about the same size as those of apes living today. Then slowly, and increasingly over the past 500,000 years, humans developed a brain that is "enormous" for an animal our size, explains Mosconi—a brain that is capable of language, complex and symbolic thought, organization and socialization, and all the other mental actions that make us truly human.

The foods that enabled our brains to grow and thrive are those our species has eaten for more than 99% of our time on Earth, a diet consumed by a people who were hunter-gatherers until the very recent past (evolutionarily speaking). It was a diet of grasses, seeds, roots, bulbs, tubers, fruits and the occasional wild-caught meat or fish—more fish than meat, Mosconi clarifies. Anthropological research reveals that meat was a rare treat for our ancestors, while fish was much easier (and less dangerous) to acquire. And fish and shellfish are excellent sources of polyunsaturated fat, including the now-famous omega-3 fatty acids that we've come to realize are super healthy. "That's the very fat that our brains are in large part made of," Mosconi points out. "Fish also contain a bounty of protein, vitamins and minerals that are essential for brain function."

If this "caveman" diet sounds familiar, that's because it echoes what up-to-the-minute science now recognizes as hands-down the healthiest menu for your brain: the Mediterranean diet. Unfortunately, though, rather than eating what our DNA is coded for, in the past century or so the industrialized world has instead been conducting what is essentially an uncontrolled dietary experiment. We eat things that people as recently as the 19th century wouldn't have even recognized as food: packaged, microwavable meals that have been stripped of their original nutrients and pumped up with artificial ingredients and flavorings; sodas that are pure high-fructose sugar; super-refined grains that spike blood sugar and can lead to diabetes and heart disease.

It's not a surprise that rates of Alzheimer's and other neurological diseases are on the rise, along with mental health issues such as anxiety and depression, and that so many of us complain of fatigue, "brain fog" or memory issues. It's because the average American's

Our brains literally developed over millennia thanks largely to a diet that emphasized healthy fats like fish.

brain is starving for the whole, unadulterated foods that originally made us who we are.

FUTURE BRAIN FOOD

The ways that different nutrients affect brain function are incredibly varied, involving inflammation, hormones, peptides, signaling molecules, cell membranes, blood vessels, neurotransmitters and many other pathways. Our bodies are like machines. And as with any machine—for example, an expensive car—the mechanisms run more smoothly, and the car lasts much longer, on superior fuel. Food is about taste, culture and celebration, but also about chemistry. "You can think of food as brain medicine," says Brizendine. "The goals are both brain integrity—retaining its size and structure as you get older—and brain plasticity, meaning to make new cells and connect more neurons."

This book will explain how the mechanisms of food nutrients play a powerful role in the three key areas of how your brain works: its cognitive power and capabilities; its moods and emotions; and its ability to remain strong throughout life, staving off mental decline. Beyond that, though, we'll celebrate the delicious foods that will drive that brain power— along with the tastiest recipes, to take advantage of their goodness.

INNER WORKINGS

* RESEARCH IS BEGINNING TO UNRAVEL THE COMPLEX RELATIONSHIP BETWEEN YOUR NUTRITION AND HOW WELL YOUR BRAIN WORKS. HERE'S WHAT WE KNOW SO FAR.

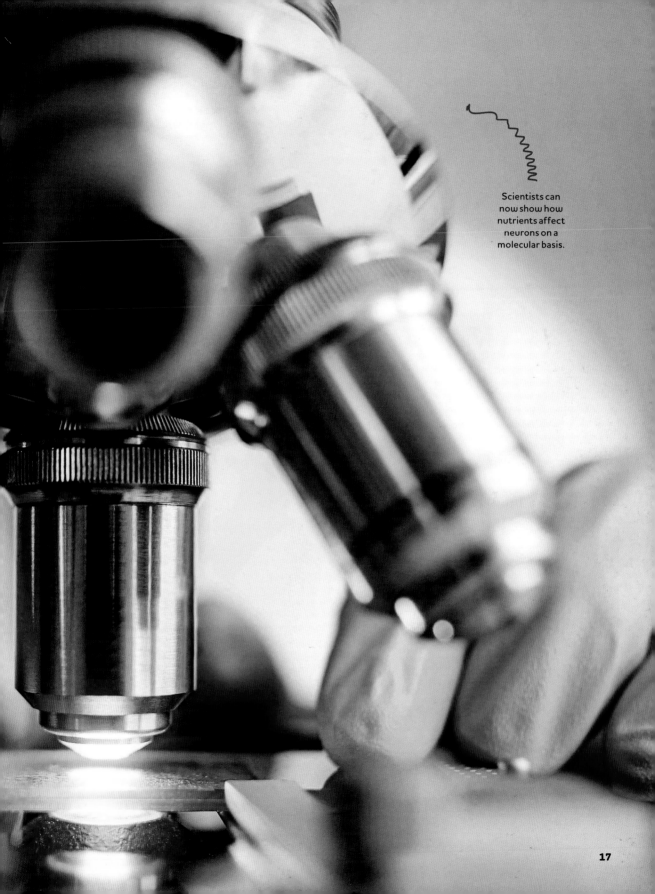

Scientists can now show how nutrients affect neurons on a molecular basis.

E at fish and broccoli, and score a stronger, better-functioning brain. Could it really be that simple? It has been easier for scientists to see the big picture—that people who follow a Mediterranean diet plan rich in seafood and plant foods have less cognitive decline and more mental agility—than to understand the *how* and *why* of that picture. Two things are becoming clear: The brain is an extremely hungry organ, demanding about one-fifth of our daily calorie intake, and it is also a vulnerable organ, capable of being damaged simply through its own day-to-day functioning. The right kinds of foods can ensure both that you take in enough nutrients to feed it with optimum ingredients and that you protect it from the ravages of daily life. Read on for an in-depth explication of the latest findings about your brain at work, and how nutrition makes it all happen.

A TOUR OF THE BRAIN

It should come as no surprise that the brain is a highly specialized organ. It is, after all, the CEO for your entire body—ensuring that your other organs and your muscles do what's necessary to keep you alive and functioning. The brain makes it possible on a moment-to-moment basis for you to breathe, move and digest, in addition to the more sophisticated activity we usually picture the brain doing: thinking. So while a dedicated part of your brain is busy with "housekeeping," controlling things like body temperature, blood pressure, and the reflexes that make you recoil from a hot stove, your thinking brain is free to plan, speak, write, concentrate, remember what happened yesterday and look forward to your summer vacation.

The "thinking" parts of the brain are in the cerebrum, and within that region the main thought-processing areas are the hippocampus (the center of memory and learning) and the amygdala (the center of emotional processing). Both are part of a larger system called the limbic system, a neural network that mediates many aspects of emotion and memory, and each has been shown to be highly affected—in both positive and negative ways—by the types of nutrients you eat.

Just one simple example out of many: Compounds in certain fruits and vegetables called flavonols, when added to the diet, have been shown to "increase hippocampus-dependent memory in mice," according to research in the journal *Nature Reviews Neuroscience*. And in a study in *Neural Regeneration Research*, anthocyanins, compounds found in berries, increased signaling between neurons in the hippocampus— and more communication means

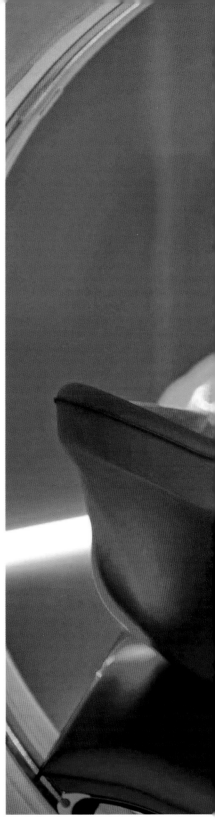

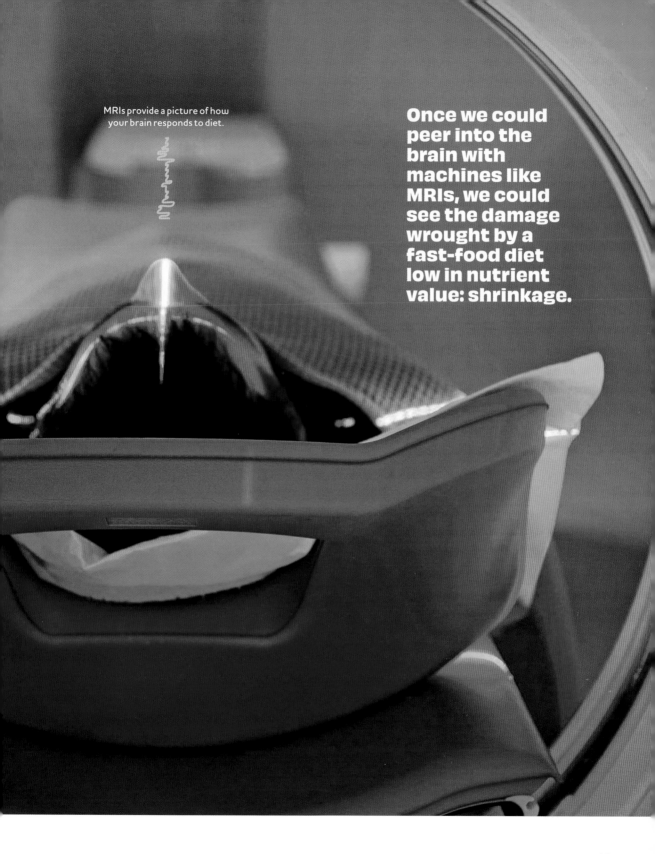

MRIs provide a picture of how your brain responds to diet.

Once we could peer into the brain with machines like MRIs, we could see the damage wrought by a fast-food diet low in nutrient value: shrinkage.

more activity and ultimately better learning and memory.

The brain is so sensitive to every substance that reaches it, in fact, that it has its own border troops, a physical barricade called the blood-brain barrier (BBB). The BBB is a wall of sorts between the brain's blood vessels and the cells and other components of brain tissue, and only "approved" entities are allowed to cross the BBB and make their way directly into the cells of the brain. Some of these, like oxygen and water, can cross the barrier freely. Others, including glucose, can cross only with help from transporter proteins, which act like special doormen that open exclusively for particular molecules, like a bouncer at a nightclub entrance.

The BBB enables the brain to protect itself from harmful substances such as bacteria and toxins, and to benefit from nutrients that are necessary for good brain function. When it was found that certain food compounds, like the anthocyanins in berries, can accumulate in the cerebral regions responsible for cognitive function, that was a sign that the brain recognizes these compounds as beneficial to cognition.

THE BRAIN'S ENEMIES

Just as the BBB protects your brain from unwelcome molecular intruders, your brain's neurons

The blood-brain barrier allows certain nutrients to pass into the brain while keeping out toxins.

themselves need defense, called neuroprotection, against various destructive forces. That's because the very acts your brain carries out every day—burning glucose and oxygen to produce energy, firing off neurons and facilitating communication across synapses, even just dealing with the normal mental and emotional stresses of life—wreak a kind of collateral damage. Many studies over the past two decades have found that nutrients in certain foods offer

just the kind of neuroprotection and healing processes the human brain needs.

First, there's the damage resulting from burning glucose for fuel, called oxidation, which produces harmful molecules known as free radicals. These injurious molecules "make their way through our neurons like little tornadoes," says neuroscientist Lisa Mosconi, PhD, associate director of the Alzheimer's Prevention Clinic at Weill Cornell Medical College/ NewYork-Presbyterian Hospital. Luckily, there is an opposing, protective force: antioxidants, substances that "wander through our bodies, including the brain, fighting off free radicals along the way," says Mosconi—like molecular police officers chasing away the bad guys. Our bodies can manufacture some

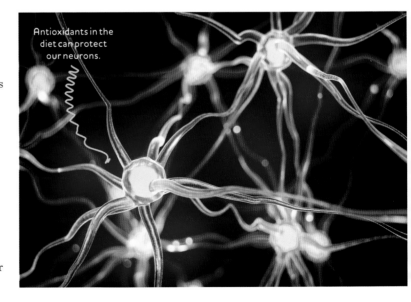

Antioxidants in the diet can protect our neurons.

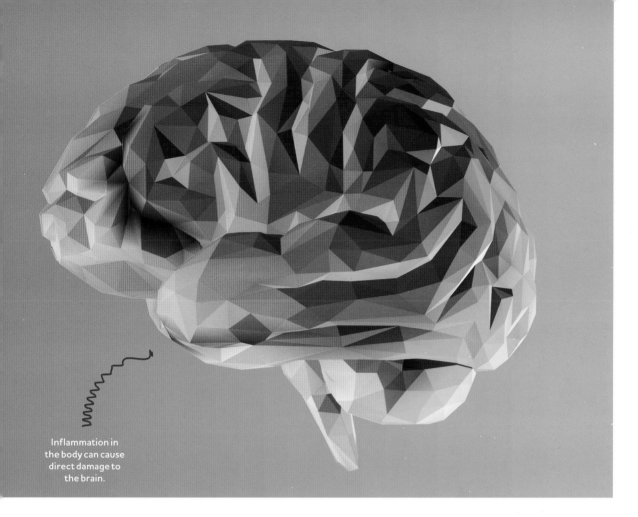

Inflammation in the body can cause direct damage to the brain.

antioxidants, but most of them come from our diets—especially from foods high in vitamin C or vitamin E. Large studies in the U.S. and elsewhere have shown a direct line between intake of these vitamins and a lower risk of developing dementia.

Other compounds in foods can fight oxidative stress as well, including the omega-3 fatty acid docosahexaenoic acid (DHA), which is present in fish, along with being the most abundant phospholipid in the human brain. A study in the journal *Current Opinion in Clinical Nutrition and Metabolic Care* found that

oxidative stress can damage cell membranes in the brain and disrupt signaling between neurons, making it harder for the brain to function properly. Researchers concluded that adding extra DHA through the diet, aka eating more of certain types of fish, "seems crucial for supporting [cell] membrane function, interneuronal signaling and cognition."

Another kind of damage our brains can cook up as an offshoot of doing its job is inflammation, a natural reaction of the immune system that can spin out of control and start destroying

neurons. Inflammation has, in recent years, been increasingly understood as a driver in all kinds of diseases, including cancer, cardiovascular disease and dementia. It can result from many different sources, including emotional stress, lack of sleep or exercise, having excess abdominal fat and, as more and more research has shown, from a diet high in sugar, unhealthy fats and processed foods.

"Inflammation is so important to health and aging that scientists are now calling it 'inflamm-aging,'" says neuropsychiatrist Louann

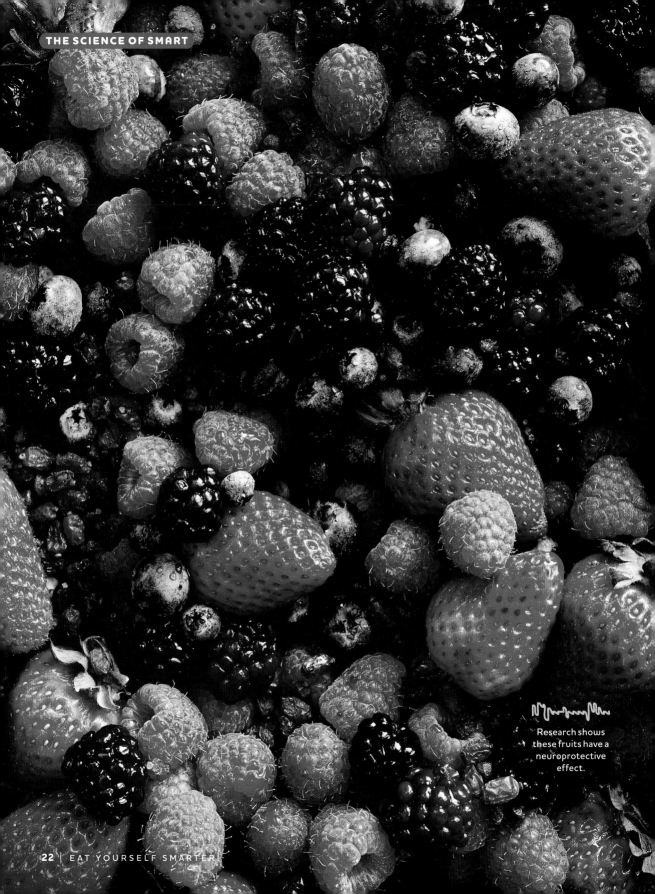

Research shows these fruits have a neuroprotective effect.

Brizendine, MD, author of *The Female Brain* and *The Male Brain*. "Chronic inflammation affects both your body and your brain on a cellular level." Studies have shown that inflammatory molecules called cytokines can disrupt the release of key neurotransmitters in the brain, and that older people with high blood levels of inflammatory markers like IL6 showed shrinkage in the brain—which is often a sign of pre-dementia. Chronic inflammation, and the overactive molecules it unleashes, can put a monkey wrench in cognitive function by disrupting the communication signals between neurons.

Here, too, food can come to the rescue. A recent comprehensive review published in the journal *Foods* found that a large group of plant micronutrients called polyphenols have a neuroprotective effect against inflammation, specifically targeting and inhibiting the action of inflammatory cytokines. One type of polyphenol in particular, called isoflavones (which are abundant in soy as well as other legumes and some fruits and nuts), can cross the blood-brain barrier to fight cytokines and quell neuroinflammation. Other studies have linked a high intake of fruits and vegetables, which are rich in a wide variety of polyphenols, to lower levels of inflammatory biomarkers in the blood.

ALL OF A PIECE

These interconnections between various foods and the way the human brain functions and protects itself make complete sense when you consider early man's diet, says Mosconi. We were hunter-gatherers who munched on whatever plants, fruits and seeds we could find, along with the occasional wild-caught fish and the very-occasional feast of wild-caught meat. Our brains evolved in concert with these foods, and many of the micronutrients in them—like omega-3 fatty acids—are building blocks within our brains themselves. So when you base your diet on these nutrients, it's like giving mother's milk to a baby: They feed and maintain our cognitive function as nature intended.

TOP 10
Inflammation Fighters

OF ALL THE THREATS YOUR BRAIN CAN FACE, CHRONIC INFLAMMATION IS ONE OF THE MOST DESTRUCTIVE. PUT THESE FOODS AT THE TOP OF YOUR MENU TO REDUCE INFLAMMATION AND HELP YOUR NEURONS COMMUNICATE WITH EACH OTHER.

FOOD	MAGIC INGREDIENT(S)
* Avocados	Potassium, magnesium, carotenoids
* Berries	Anthocyanins
* Broccoli	Sulforaphane
* Dark Chocolate	Flavanols
* Fatty Fish	Omega-3 fatty acids
* Grapes	Anthocyanins, resveratrol
* Green Tea	EGCG (epigallocatechin-3-gallate)
* Peppers	Quercetin, vitamin C
* Tomatoes	Lycopene, potassium, vitamin C
* Turmeric	Curcumin

Gut Instincts

★ YOUR DIET HAS A POWERFUL IMPACT ON YOUR DIGESTIVE SYSTEM'S MICROBIOME—WHICH, EMERGING RESEARCH SUGGESTS, MAY AFFECT MOOD, MEMORY AND AGING.

If you've ever been on a date and felt your stomach flip-flopping, or gotten a little queasy before a big presentation, you should have an inkling that the thoughts running through your brain can have a very real impact on what's happening in your gut.

But this link is far more powerful than most people realize, and, perhaps most surprisingly, it's not a one-way street: Yes, your mood has the potential to impact the inner workings of your GI tract, but your digestive system—and the foods you put into it—also have the ability to influence your mental state, memory and thought processes.

Exactly how this occurs is an area of emerging research, but it's clear that the main connector is the vagus nerve. A neuron-rich superhighway, the vagus nerve starts in the brain and runs down through the neck and abdomen, all the way to the colon. It regulates many bodily functions that you never have to think about, including respiration and heart rate. It also serves as a physical link between the brain in your head and the "second brain" in your gut, a pathway that scientists refer to as the brain-gut axis.

Yes, that's right—you have another brain in your gut, and the vagus nerve connects it to the main brain in your head. The second brain, which is officially called the enteric nervous system, is comprised of millions of interconnected nerve cells that are wrapped around the bulk of your digestive tract. There is another important team of players in your digestive system, though, and they outnumber even your nerve cells. It is estimated that as many as a trillion microorganisms, both good and bad, inhabit your gut. Collectively known as the gut microbiome, they're fueled by the foods you eat, and studies are showing they may have an outsize effect on brain function, emotions and possibly even the risk of developing dementia as you age.

Your body's "second brain"
in your gut can have a
significant influence
on your health.

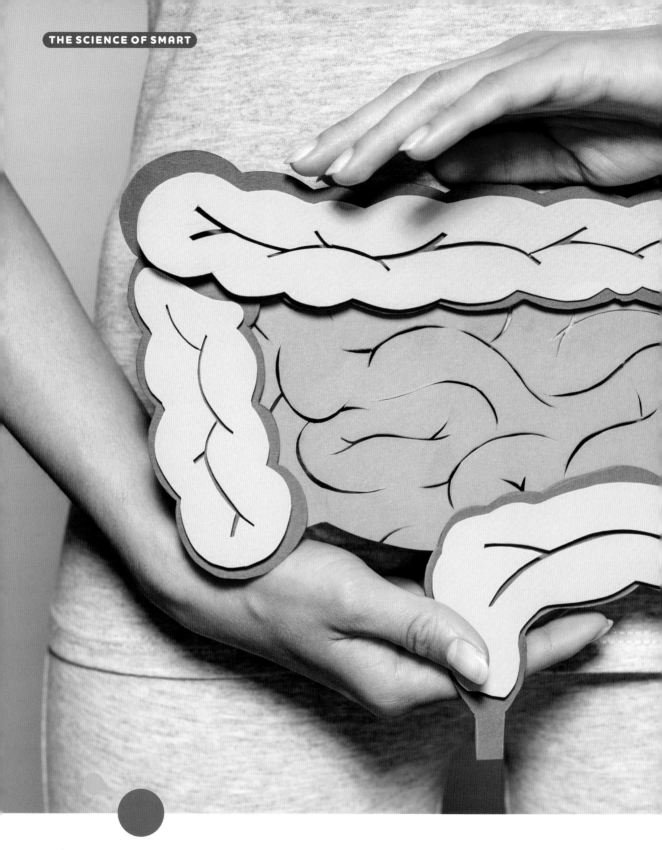

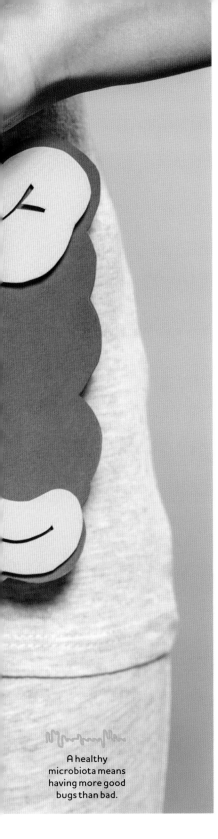

A healthy microbiota means having more good bugs than bad.

HOW THE SECOND BRAIN WORKS

Unlike the big brain in your head, the little brain in your gut doesn't feel emotions, doesn't process life lessons and isn't capable of higher-level decision-making. Its chief job, says Emeran Mayer, MD, a distinguished research professor at UCLA's Division of Digestive Diseases and director of the G. Oppenheimer Center for Neurobiology of Stress and Resilience, is to operate the gastrointestinal system—and it doesn't need any help from the big brain to do that.

"Everything that goes on in the gut—contractions, secretion of fluids, blood flow—is essentially regulated by that second brain," says Mayer, author of *The Mind-Gut Connection* and *The Gut-Immune Connection*. From an evolutionary perspective, this gut-based brain actually precedes the big brain, Mayer adds. Over time, as animals advanced, the more complex organ in our heads developed, and it uses most of the same neurotransmitters (chemical messengers) as the gut brain.

What this means is that these two seemingly disparate body parts—your brain and your gut—have the tools and means to regularly "talk" to each other. Even better, you have the power to influence that conversation by changing your diet.

Making better diet choices can turn up immune function in the gut while also reducing inflammation everywhere.

GOOD (AND BAD) BUGS

Depression and anxiety, whether formally diagnosed or not, are incredibly common. Memory issues, including Alzheimer's disease and other forms of dementia, are also quite prevalent. These problems are multifaceted and likely arise due to some combination of inherited predisposition and environmental influence— perhaps including the foods you put in your mouth.

No one is saying that you can prevent depression or ward off Alzheimer's simply by eating more salads. But emerging research does suggest that altering your diet can tame overactive immune cells in your gut and, in turn, ease low-grade brain inflammation, reducing your risk of a variety of mood and cognitive issues.

In order for this to happen, you have to change your microbiota— that vast universe of bacteria, viruses, fungi and other organisms living in your digestive tract. Some of these

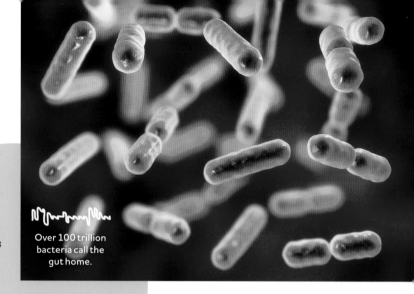

Over 100 trillion bacteria call the gut home.

organisms are beneficial and others are harmful; when you have enough "good" bacteria and other organisms to keep the troublesome ones in check, inflammation in the gut goes down. In one study published in the *Journal of Neuroinflammation*, researchers from China and the U.S. found evidence of a relationship between the composition of the gut microbiota and Alzheimer's disease, major depression and schizophrenia.

"'Good' bacteria may generate small molecules, like metabolites [byproducts], that may be beneficial to brain health and delay the development of dementia," says study co-author Lu Qi, MD, PhD, director of the Tulane University Obesity Research Center and adjunct professor of nutrition at Harvard T.H. Chan School of Public Health. These byproducts include gamma-Aminobutyric acid (GABA) and serotonin, two mood chemicals that are

Half an avocado spread on a piece of whole-wheat toast can supply one-third of the daily fiber you need—which will make your gut bacteria happy.

associated with feelings of calmness and relaxation.

Mayer, who has long studied the gut-brain connection, says that many studies have hinted at the close relationship between the microbiota and emotional health. He notes that scientists have actually manipulated the microbiota of mice in such a way that it caused the animals to exhibit new signs of depression. "This is more difficult to demonstrate in humans, but a recent Spanish study did show that people on antidepressant medication who ate a traditional Mediterranean diet fared better" than those who were following the typical Western diet.

CHOOSING A GUT-HEALTHY DIET

What's so special about the Mediterranean diet? For starters, it's 75% plant-based, so it's rich in fiber and polyphenols, a specific type of antioxidant that gets broken down in the gut into smaller, health-promoting molecules.

"People who eat a largely plant-based diet have a thicker and healthier mucus layer in the gut, which serves as a barrier that prevents microbes from coming into contact with immune cells in the gut wall," says Mayer. Without that barrier, immune cells get activated, which can lead to digestive distress. Low-grade inflammation in the gut may also spill over into the bloodstream and travel to any organ—including the brain.

"If this happens on a chronic basis, it can activate immune cells in the brain and you end up with inflammatory cytokines [proteins] floating around and influencing nerve cells in the brain," Mayer continues. "That might feel like 'brain fog' or fatigue or trouble concentrating, but if it persists for a long time it can lead to the breakdown of nerve cells and deposits of tangles and plaques, which are manifestations of neurodegeneration" that have been associated with Alzheimer's disease.

Bile acids are likely another piece of the puzzle. These acids are naturally secreted when you eat fatty foods, so people who follow a plant-based diet (which tends to be lower in fat) have fewer of them, compared to those who eat a lot of meat. When bile acids get broken down in the gut, they turn into "secondary" bile acids, which can travel to the brain. "Secondary bile acids produced by the gut microbiota have been found in the brains of people who have died from Alzheimer's disease," says Mayer.

Another key component of the Mediterranean diet is fish, especially wild salmon, sardines and anchovies. These are rich in omega-3 fatty acids, which are well-known for lowering inflammation and promoting better physical and mental health. One recent study, in *Translational Psychiatry*, found that omega-3s may ease depression. Other studies have suggested that they may be beneficial for brain health, and

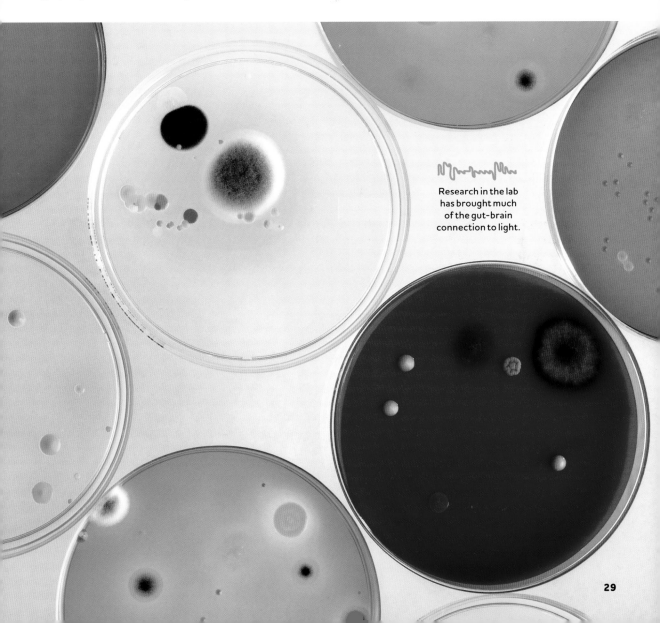

Research in the lab has brought much of the gut-brain connection to light.

some have found lower levels of certain omega-3s in the blood of people with Alzheimer's.

If you need yet another reason to choose fish over meat, consider that meat contains a nutrient that gut bacteria break down into a substance called TMA (trimethylamine), which gets further converted to TMAO (TMA plus oxide) in the liver. "TMAO has been found to worsen many health outcomes," including heart disease, says Lu, and has been linked to higher incidence of depression in some.

While overhauling your diet might seem like a lot of work, Mayer believes it's worth it. And studies have shown that the payoff kicks in quickly. "We can see improvements in inflammatory markers and gut microbes in as little as four weeks," he says—though of course you'll have to stick with your new eating plan long term if you want to reap lasting perks.

THE FIBER FACTOR

Plant-based diets are healthy for myriad reasons, but one major player is fiber, which are the parts of plant foods your body can't digest or absorb. Fiber is what fuels the good microbes in your gut: Bacteria break down fiber into beneficial chemical compounds that are sent to the brain through the bloodstream or carried as nerve signals via the vagus nerve, says neurobiology expert Emeran Mayer, MD. Those healthy compounds include butyrate, a short-chain fatty acid that promotes good digestive health and helps tame inflammation throughout the body.

HOW MUCH OF IT IS ENOUGH?

For overall good health, 25 to 38 grams per day is recommended—yet most Americans only get about 16 grams per day. Boost your digestive health by eating more leafy greens, artichokes, asparagus, berries, tomatoes and bananas; all are good sources of *prebiotics*, a specific type of plant fiber that makes it past your digestive enzymes and gets broken down by the good bacteria in the lower GI tract. Legumes and whole grains such as oats, barley and whole wheat are also good picks.

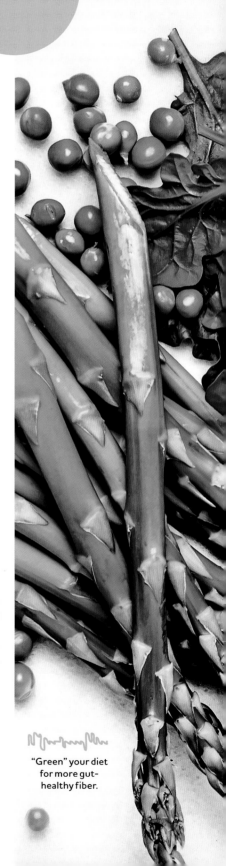

"Green" your diet for more gut-healthy fiber.

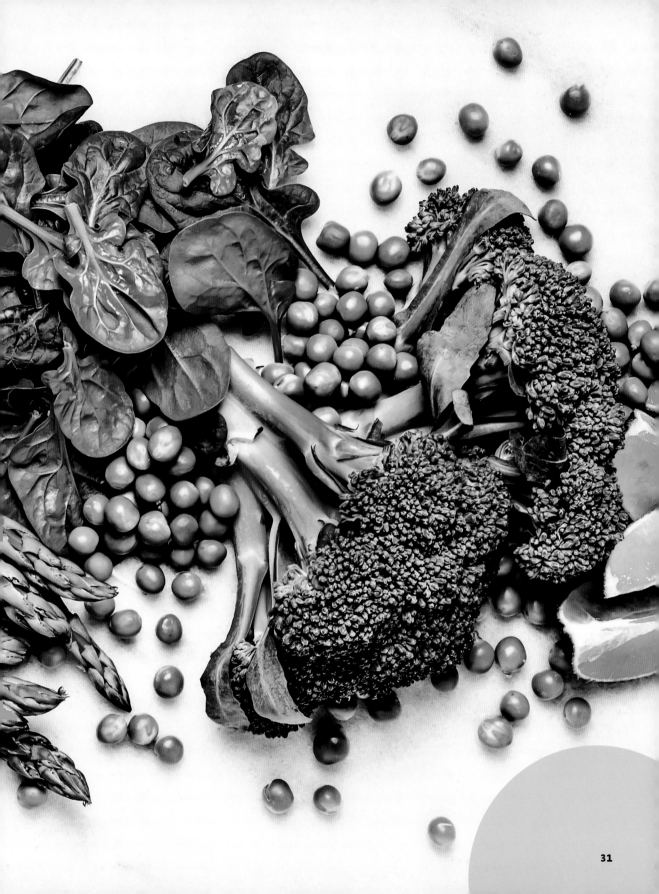

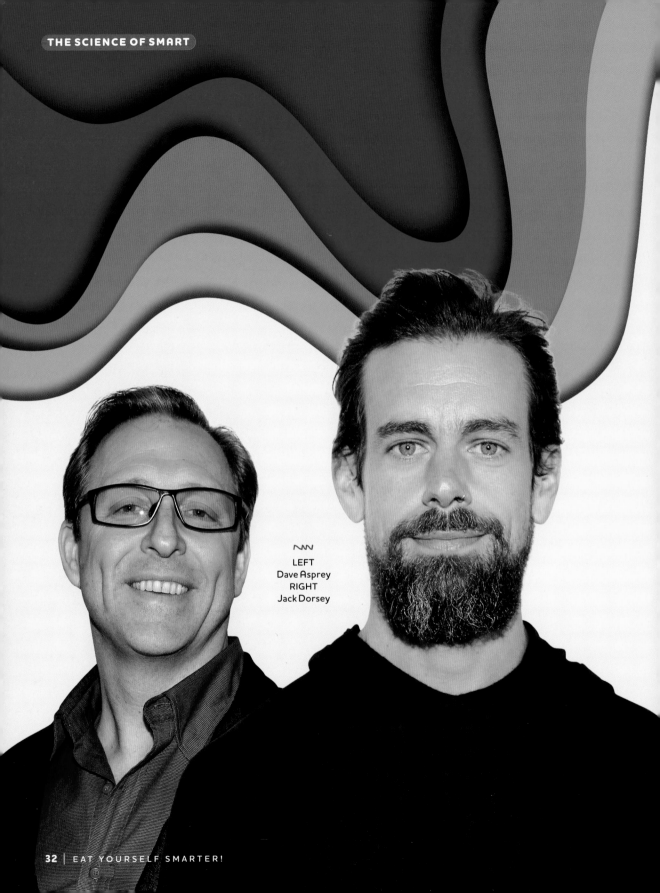

LEFT
Dave Asprey
RIGHT
Jack Dorsey

The High-Tech Brain

* CAN YOU "BIOHACK" YOUR WAY TO BETTER COGNITION? IN A WORLD HUNGRY FOR THE NEXT BIG THING IN DIET AND WELL-BEING, THE BRAINIACS IN SILICON VALLEY HAVE SOME INTRIGUING SUGGESTIONS.

Anyone obsessed with health, beauty and anti-aging has traditionally turned to Hollywood stars like Gwyneth Paltrow and Jennifer Aniston (and their celebrity trainers and nutritionists) for the latest news in diet and exercise. But that's been changing in recent years, thanks to some billionaire Silicon Valley leaders who are expanding their tech footprint to encompass health and wellness. Coining the phrase biohacking—a form of tracking and changing your body's biology through various experiments—these achievement-oriented computer scientists are using their own bodies like a research lab to enhance their physical and mental performance.

The self-proclaimed father of biohacking is tech mogul Dave Asprey, a formerly overweight self-described nerd who, fed up with his unhealthy lifestyle, deduced that, "if I can hack the internet, then I can hack my own body." To jump-start his new resolve, in 2004 he left home to travel to the Himalayas, learn meditation and hike the mountains, where he discovered the magical combination of butter and caffeine in the yak-butter teas of the region. "Five minutes after I drank it," he says on his website, bulletproof.com, "my brain fog disappeared and I felt better than I had in a long time."

When he returned to the United States, he spent years testing various combinations of butter and tea, finally settling on good old-fashioned java, which was the genesis of Bulletproof Coffee. "Not only did it taste amazing," explains Asprey, "but it turned my brain on." He lost weight, got claims his IQ went up 20 points. Soon Asprey quit the Silicon Valley grind to concentrate on coffee and start the lifestyle brand Bulletproof 360, which sells mold-free coffee beans, protein bars, MCT oil and various supplements. Nowadays, his regimen includes a morning Bulletproof coffee, followed by a diet that is high in fat, moderate in protein and low in carbs, similar to two OGs of these regimens: the Atkins Diet and keto.

And if you're skeptical about his increased brain-power brags, get this: He's since written six books—four of them bestsellers, including the latest,

Some Silicon Valley titans expound the benefits of fasting as a way to increase both energy and focus.

Fast This Way: Burn Fat, Heal Inflammation, and Eat Like the High Performing Human You Were Meant to Be. He's also the host of a top health podcast, called Bulletproof Radio, *and* says he plans to live to be 180.

Another founding father of the biohack movement is Jack Dorsey, the smart but somewhat quirky CEO of the billion dollar-valued companies Twitter and Square. With the stress of his two huge jobs, Dorsey seems to be willing to try almost anything to improve his physical and mental agility. As he explained on the podcast The Boardroom: Out of the Office, "I got super-serious about meditation and really serious about dedicating a lot more of my time and energy to working out and staying physically healthy and looking more critically at my diet. I had to, just to stay above water."

Dorsey famously wakes up at 5 a.m. to meditate for two hours, then drinks a glass of his "salt juice" ($^1/_4$ teaspoon Himalayan salt, a squeeze of half a lemon, and 12 ounces of water). Since he is a fan of extreme intermittent fasting, including dopamine fasts (more on those later), he claims salt juice hydrates the body during a fast and replaces electrolytes. After the "juice," he walks 5 miles to his office, where he's such a juice booster that all of his 4,500 employees are given a glass of it every morning. To make sure his body stays on track, he also had a blood glucose monitor implanted in his body to measure the amount of sugar in his blood.

If you think these two influential geniuses are the exception in these eccentric lifestyle choices, think again. Many tech types—and many of them male—experiment with diet, fasting, meditation and exercise to stay lean, energized and focused. And not only are they encouraging their thousands of employees to embrace their methods, they've also got millions of social media followers who hang on their every tweet to glean their newest health hacks. "Mr. Dorsey's a successful guy,"

Bulletproof plans center on coffee amped up with a dose of fat.

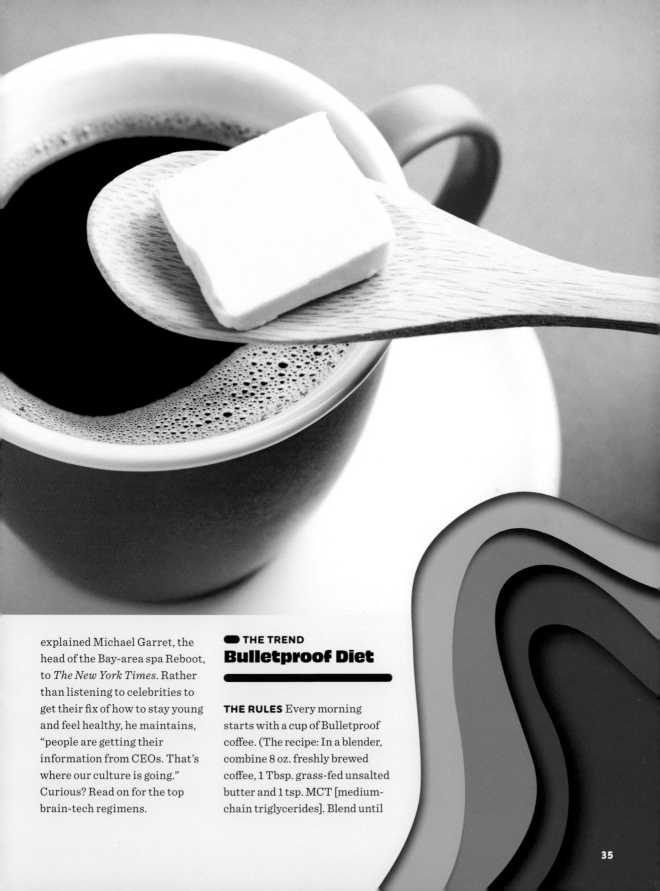

explained Michael Garret, the head of the Bay-area spa Reboot, to *The New York Times*. Rather than listening to celebrities to get their fix of how to stay young and feel healthy, he maintains, "people are getting their information from CEOs. That's where our culture is going." Curious? Read on for the top brain-tech regimens.

THE TREND
Bulletproof Diet

THE RULES Every morning starts with a cup of Bulletproof coffee. (The recipe: In a blender, combine 8 oz. freshly brewed coffee, 1 Tbsp. grass-fed unsalted butter and 1 tsp. MCT [medium-chain triglycerides]. Blend until frothy.) This amped-up brew is said to suppress hunger and boost mental clarity.

The regimen Asprey developed is not just about the java, though: It includes a diet that is high fat, moderate in protein and very low in carbs. In fact, it's essentially modified keto, with an emphasis on lots of brain-friendly veggies, along with some carb "refeed" days where foods such as sweet potatoes and squash are on the menu.

THE SCIENCE Coffee is linked to many health benefits, including reducing the risk of diabetes, cancer and heart disease, and MCT oil has been shown to reduce appetite and boost metabolism. A keto-like diet appears to have benefits as well (read on for more).

THE RESULTS The Bulletproof diet can help your body go into ketosis, which may trigger weight loss and improve cognition, but it can feel restrictive.

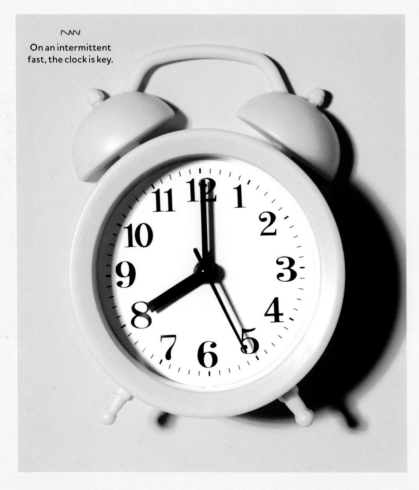

On an intermittent fast, the clock is key.

THE TREND
Intermittent Fasting

THE RULES An ancient practice that has become one of the most popular regimens on the planet, IF involves going for periods of time without food, ranging from not eating for eight hours every day to making two or more days per week very-low-calorie. Dorsey practices IF on the extreme end, eating one meal a day (called OMAD) and then fasting completely all weekend (some have called this a form of disordered eating, but Dorsey swears by it for high mental performance).

THE SCIENCE When you fast, insulin levels drop, initiating fat-burning; human growth hormone increases, which also helps with fat burning and muscle gain; cellular repair increases; and studies have shown that fasting may promote neuroplasticity.

THE RESULTS Weight loss, especially in the belly; increased metabolism; a lower risk of type 2 diabetes and heart disease; a reduction in inflammation throughout the body.

THE TREND
Keto

THE RULES High fat/low carb eating plan. And if you combine

How the Brightest Feed Their Brains

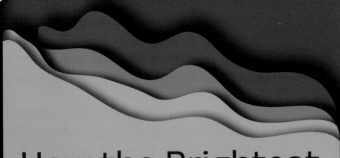

WHAT'S THE SECRET? THESE SUPER-SUCCESSFUL PEOPLE EACH HAVE THEIR OWN FORMULA.

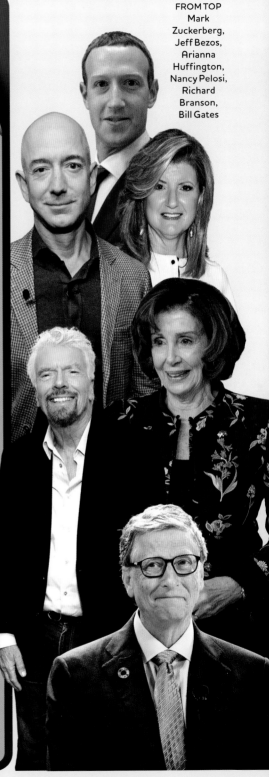

MARK ZUCKERBERG

For years, the Facebook founder was a vegetarian, taking advantage of brain-boosting plant foods. In 2011 he began eating meat again—but only if he had killed the animal himself. Now he eats some meat, but he leaves the slaughtering to the pros.

JEFF BEZOS

The richest man in history is known for adventurous food choices: Bezos was once photographed eating iguana, and at a high-profile breakfast meeting he famously ordered octopus with potatoes, bacon, green-garlic yogurt and eggs. His real secret weapon: at least eight hours of solid shut-eye nightly.

ARIANNA HUFFINGTON

The media mogul told CNN her morning meal consists of "fresh fruit, poached eggs and two hot cups of Bulletproof coffee."

RICHARD BRANSON

So very British: The founder of venture capital conglomerate The Virgin Group estimates he drinks 20 cups of tea a day.

NANCY PELOSI

The Speaker of the U.S. House of Representatives, Pelosi told *Food & Wine* that she has eaten dark chocolate ice cream for breakfast daily for years. "I don't see it as different from a cup of coffee," she said.

BILL GATES

The billionaire philanthropist and Microsoft co-founder has said he loves Diet Coke so much that he drinks multiple cans a day. Though caffeine is linked to increased alertness and mental performance, diet soda isn't the healthiest delivery system.

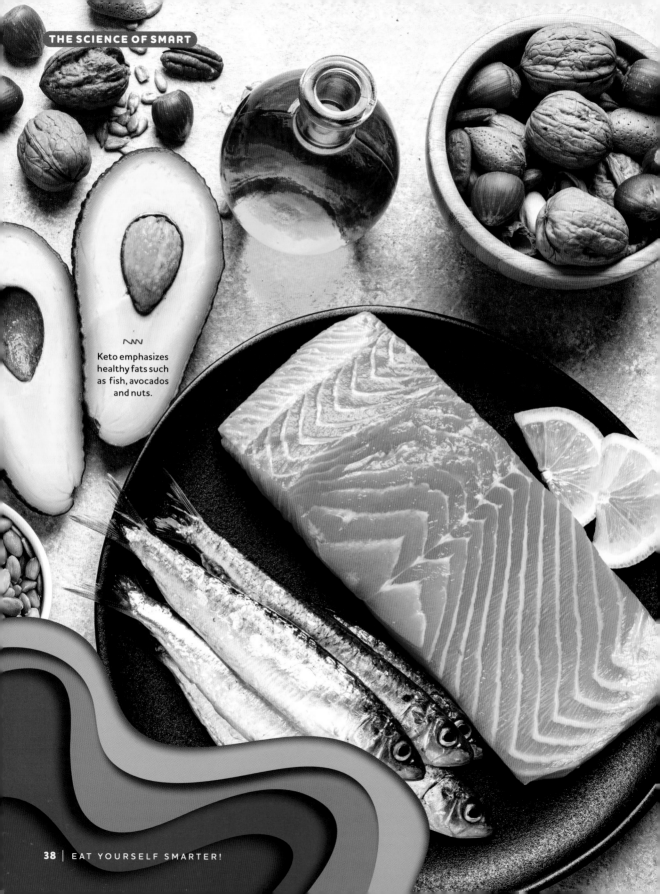

Keto emphasizes healthy fats such as fish, avocados and nuts.

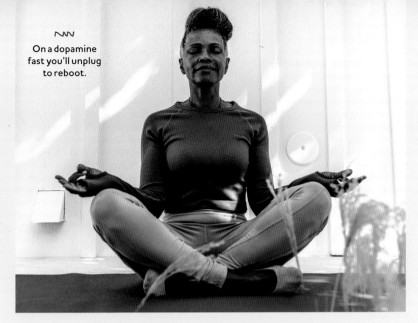

On a dopamine fast you'll unplug to reboot.

it with intermittent fasting, that may be even better.

THE SCIENCE Research shows brain cells may work more efficiently when they run on ketones for fuel rather than glucose. Ketones are made from fat, so when you are in the state of ketosis, your body is burning fat instead of sugar.

THE RESULTS Less brain fog; improved cognition and memory in older adults with risks of Alzheimer's, and those with epilepsy, autism and Parkinson's disease; more sustained energy with no afternoon crashes; reduced appetite; weight loss. Its fans include many NoCal tech geeks who use it to "downsize" their waistline.

 THE TREND
Dopamine Fasts

THE RULES No food, no sex, no alcohol, no screens, no music, no talking, no fun! This plan, created by Cameron Sepah, PhD, assistant clinical professor of neuroscience at UCSF Medical School and start-up investor, can be for one day every month, or more often. Popular time periods are 24 to 48 hours. You spend the downtime fasting, doing yoga, meditating, walking in a quiet neighborhood, remaining silent.
THE SCIENCE Quite simply, by eliminating almost all normal everyday stimuli and/or detoxing

from problematic behavior, you allow your neurotransmitters and receptors to calm down and the brain to reset.
THE RESULTS According to followers, after a dopamine fast they feel more focused and find more joy in the activities they had taken a break from.

THE TREND
Soylent

THE RULES There are four types of these products that were developed by Rob Rhinehart, a software engineer and the

How does Soylent taste? "Like I would expect day-old pancake batter to taste," wrote one reviewer.

company's founder: bottled Soylent drinks; Soylent Powder, to make shakes; Soylent Stacked, a caffeine-packed formula that will kick-start your body and brain; and Soylent Squared, 100-calorie nutrition bars.
THE SCIENCE Soylent is made from soybeans, which contain the most complete plant-based source of protein; 39 essential nutrients, including healthy fats, vitamins, minerals, fatty acids and amino acids for that satiated feeling; and allulose, a low-calorie carb that doesn't raise insulin levels. Each drink contains 400 calories.
THE RESULTS The original goal was to create nutritional meals on-the-go so techies could work through their lunches and dinners. If you drink five a day, you're taking in 2,000 calories, so weight loss may be minimal. Some consumers say they feel better and more energized; others complain that it takes the pleasure out of eating.

Get SMART

⋆ **THE GOAL: STRONG CONCENTRATION, SHARP MEMORY AND SUPERIOR REASONING. READ THE INSIDE STORY OF HOW THE RIGHT FOODS CAN MAKE IT HAPPEN.**

On its face, perhaps it's not surprising that "clean," fresh foods such as asparagus and fish can make your brain work better. Certain foods, after all, are widely understood to be healthy for your body in general. But how do they affect your thinking processes, exactly? And can building your diet around fruits, vegetables, fish, nuts and healthy fats actually help you reason better, solve problems more quickly, and remember details that contribute to complex calculations? Years of research in both animals and humans, and encompassing behavioral evidence as well as brain scans, suggest that there is indeed a straight line between food and

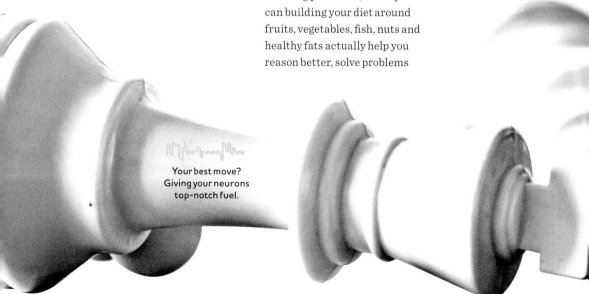

Your best move?
Giving your neurons
top-notch fuel.

cognition—and scientists are beginning to understand the mechanisms behind that process.

These mechanisms work at chemical and molecular levels to affect the way brain cells function and communicate, and point the way to honing your own thinking abilities to a finer edge. Many of these processes involve how your brain obtains the energy it needs to fuel its work, says Gary E. Gibson, PhD, director of the Laboratory for Mitochondrial Biology and Metabolic Dysfunction in Neurodegeneration at the Burke Neurological Institute. That's because "the brain consumes an immense amount of energy relative to the rest of the body. So the mechanisms

The brain has been shown to actually burn more calories when thinking "hard" than when vegging out.

that are involved in the transfer of energy from foods to neurons are likely to be fundamental to the control of brain function." If these mechanisms are working at their best, your brain gets the fuel it craves to figure out a logic problem or retrieve a memory. What makes these fueling mechanisms perform well? Certain nutrients, naturally.

If that sounds circular, it simply points up how central nutrition is to firing up your neurons. Here's the lowdown on the major players—both nutritionally and within the brain's structure—in the all-important job of thinking clearly and incisively.

NEUROGENESIS AND PLASTICITY

What's better for cognition than having a lot of brain cells? Making even *more* brain cells. That's why scientists

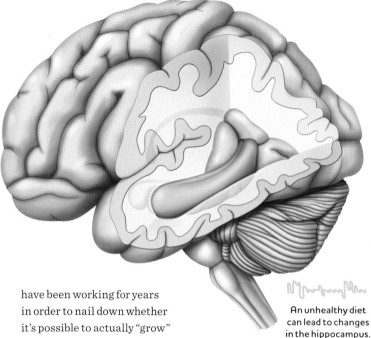

An unhealthy diet can lead to changes in the hippocampus.

have been working for years in order to nail down whether it's possible to actually "grow" new brain cells, or neurons, a process called neurogenesis. Until a few decades ago most neuroscientists thought we were born with all the neurons we would ever have, according to the National Institutes of Health. Since the 1960s, though, increasing evidence has pointed to neurogenesis being real— although the concept still has believers on both sides.

A small 2018 study in the journal *Nature* found no "immature neurons" in any of the 29 adult brains that researchers examined, but the results were hotly contested by other scientists. Meanwhile, many neuroscientists are convinced that neurogenesis is possible, and that food (as well as exercise) can play an important role. A study in the journal *Advances in Nutrition* in 2017 proposed that "many

dietary components such as curcumin, resveratrol, blueberry polyphenols, sulforaphane, salvianolic acid, polyunsaturated fatty acids (PUFAs), and diets enriched with polyphenols and PUFAs...induce neurogenesis in adult brains."

Translation to foods? Those components are present in the

Researchers have called the brain an "expensive organ" because of its high demand for fuel, relative to the rest of the body (yes, even the muscles!).

spice turmeric, grapes, red wine, blueberries, cranberries, dark chocolate, broccoli, omega-3 fatty acids and a slew of other fruits and vegetables rich in polyphenols.

Another study, in the journal *Foods* in 2019, called neurogenesis "a crucial factor in preserving cognitive function and repairing damaged brain cells affected by aging and brain disorders." And, most promising, the study found that diets rich in polyphenols have been shown to induce that neurogenesis "in the hippocampal region," the memory-and-learning part of the brain.

More brain cells mean not only simply more capacity but more communication, more opportunities for neurons to pass along information—like that memory you're trying to retrieve for a project you're working on. That's where a phenomenon called neuroplasticity comes in, which works hand in hand with neurogenesis.

Neuroplasticity is the ability of the brain to change its wiring to work better. It literally means transforming the way that synapses (the little spaces between neurons that transfer messages from one cell to the next) pass along signals. It's basically a microcosm of the learning process: Your brain is constantly "pruning" itself, getting rid of those neural connections that aren't being used while strengthening

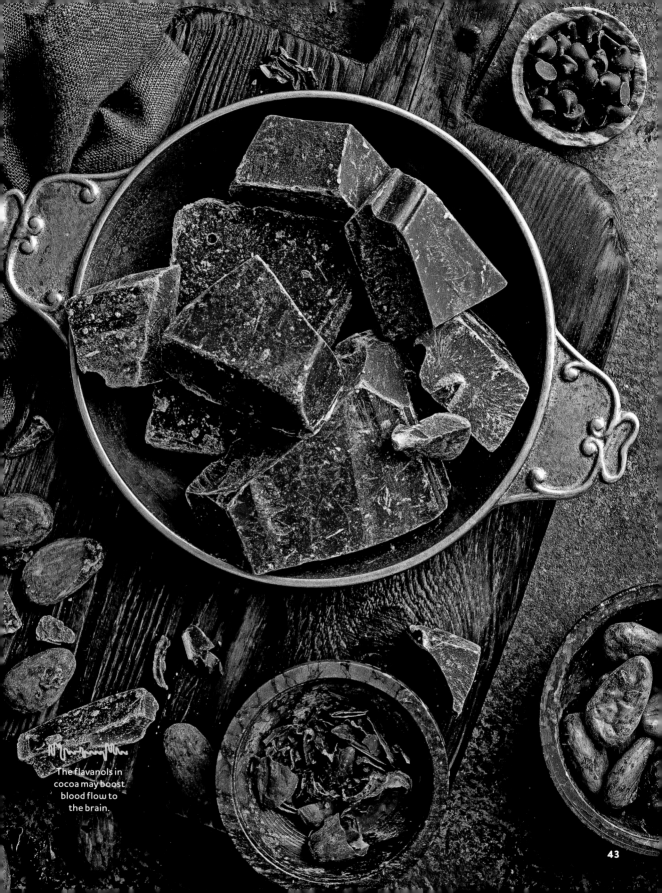

The flavanols in cocoa may boost blood flow to the brain.

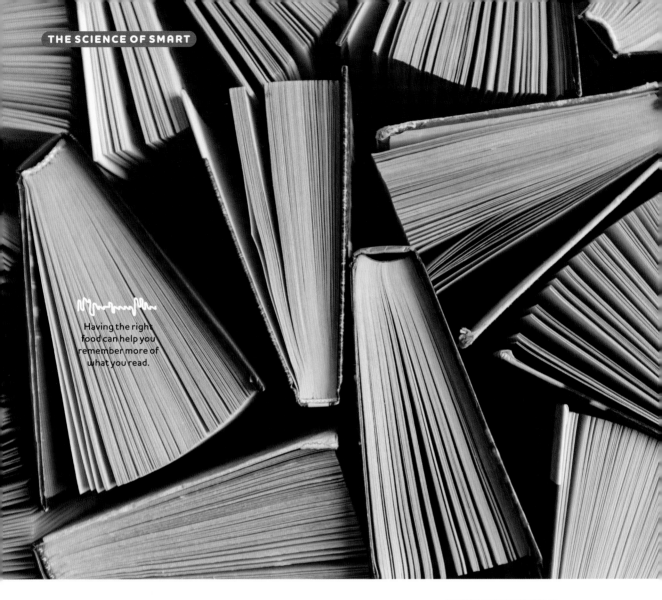

Having the right food can help you remember more of what you read.

others. Plasticity is your brain getting smarter, and certain foods can help—or hinder—this rewiring process.

For instance, studies have found that a high-sugar diet can decrease neuroplasticity, while a diet rich in certain compounds can foster plasticity. According to the *Advances in Nutrition* study, these include many of the compounds that also promote neurogenesis:

folic acid, vitamin E, omega-3 fatty acids and "polyphenols found in fruits, vegetables, nuts and spices." Still, how does this come about, and why do these foods make your neurons smarter? For that, you need to look to Gibson's description of the mechanisms that actually transfer energy from foods to the brain—metabolism—and the host of chemical aides that make it happen.

THE HELPERS

Neurons may be the building blocks of the brain, the cells that make up the actual gray matter, but they rely on an army of other substances that act as intermediaries in supplying them with food. Picture a group of grocery-store deliverymen: neurotransmitters with names such as norepinephrine and serotonin, and proteins like brain-derived neurotrophic factor (BDNF). BDNF is a multitasker, having emerged as a major player in both metabolizing food compounds (that is, breaking them down for use as energy in the brain) and increasing neuroplasticity.

A study in the journal *Current Opinion in Clinical Nutrition and Metabolic Care* found that BDNF acts as a mediator in the process of delivering energy to "cognitive centers such as the hippocampus." The study describes "the several roles of BDNF on cognition and emotions," including boosting plasticity. Basically, the more BDNF you have circulating in your brain, the more your neurons can grow and communicate. And what raises levels of BDNF? Certain food compounds, of course, including omega-3 fatty acids and polyphenols.

Other factors that decrease neuroplasticity and slow down your brain's cognitive processes include inflammation and oxidation, and here, too, polyphenols from fruits and vegetables can come to the rescue, acting as a protective "clean-up in aisle six" battalion. Oxidation, a natural byproduct of your brain simply doing its work, produces free radicals, waste products that can gum up your thought processes (picture "brain fog"). Free radicals are destructive particles in the

5 Choices That Spike Creativity

THOUGH THE SPARK OF GENIUS MAY BE HARD TO ATTRIBUTE TO WHAT YOU EAT, THERE ARE SOME FOODS THAT SEEM TO HELP WHEN IT COMES TO GETTING THOSE JUICES FLOWING. HERE ARE A HANDFUL THAT MAY HELP YOU CHANNEL YOUR INNER ARTIST, AUTHOR OR INVENTOR.

BANANAS A study published in the journal *Psychological Research* found foods high in tyrosine (like this fruit favorite) can help drive creativity by promoting convergent ("deep") thinking. Another study in the *British Journal of Health Psychology* found that eating fruits (like bananas) and veggies was linked to an increased sense of curiosity and creativity.

EGGS The yellow stuff inside an egg is all it's cracked up to be. Yolks have both healthy fats to improve cognition and choline, which helps form acetylcholine—the neurotransmitter that plays a crucial role in memory, mood and processing speed.

GREEN TEA If you need to spur your imagination, try pouring a steaming cup of this beverage. In addition to powerful antioxidants, green tea has both caffeine to get you energized and the amino acid L-theanine, which seems to help strengthen memory and attention while boosting mood.

MACKEREL Holy you-know-what! Salmon may get all the love, but this small, fatty fish has nearly just as much omega-3s, which helps to increase connections between brain cells to get your gray matter turning.

PUMPKIN SEEDS These small snacks pack a big punch, especially when it comes to minerals like zinc, which is key for critical thinking and cognition. They're also a mood-booster thanks to their high levels of magnesium, B vitamins and tryptophan.

brain, but they can be neutralized by various compounds found in foods, including curcumin (found in turmeric), resveratrol (berries, grapes and red wine) and isoflavones (legumes, nuts, soybeans and some fruits).

Similarly, inflammation can disrupt your brain's functioning, and anti-inflammatory compounds found in berries, fish, broccoli, avocados, green tea and many other foods can actively work to calm inflammation. The result: more plasticity, less brain fog and faster mental processing times, on everything from the daily crossword to the most complex of mental gymnastics.

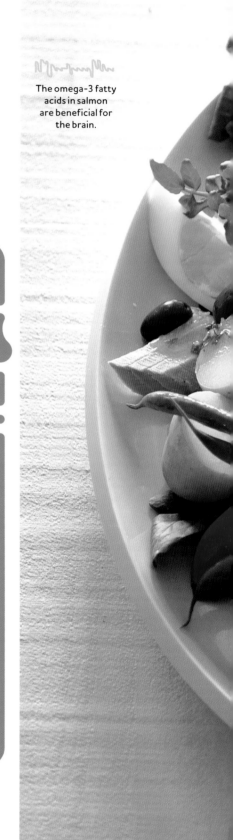

The omega-3 fatty acids in salmon are beneficial for the brain.

Food for Thought

HAVE A DAY STACKED WITH MENTAL TASKS AND A TO-DO LIST AS LONG AS YOUR ARM? TRY THIS GOOD-BRAIN-DAY EATING PLAN:

BREAKFAST 2 scrambled eggs, a side of berries, a cup of coffee
Brain Ingredients choline, anthocyanins and other antioxidants and anti-inflammatories, caffeine

LUNCH niçoise salad on a bed of greens with tuna, green beans, olives, tomatoes, olive oil dressing
Brain Ingredients polyphenols, lycopene, omega-3 fatty acids, vitamins E and K, monounsaturated fats

SNACK handful of walnuts, sunflower seeds or almonds, cup of green tea
Brain Ingredients omega-3 fatty acids, vitamin E, polyphenols, L-theanine

DINNER 6-ounce skirt steak, broccoli, baked sweet potato, 1 glass red wine
Brain Ingredients iron, vitamin B12, sulforaphane, vitamin K, carotenoids, resveratrol

THROUGHOUT THE DAY 8 glasses of water (a total of 64 ounces daily)

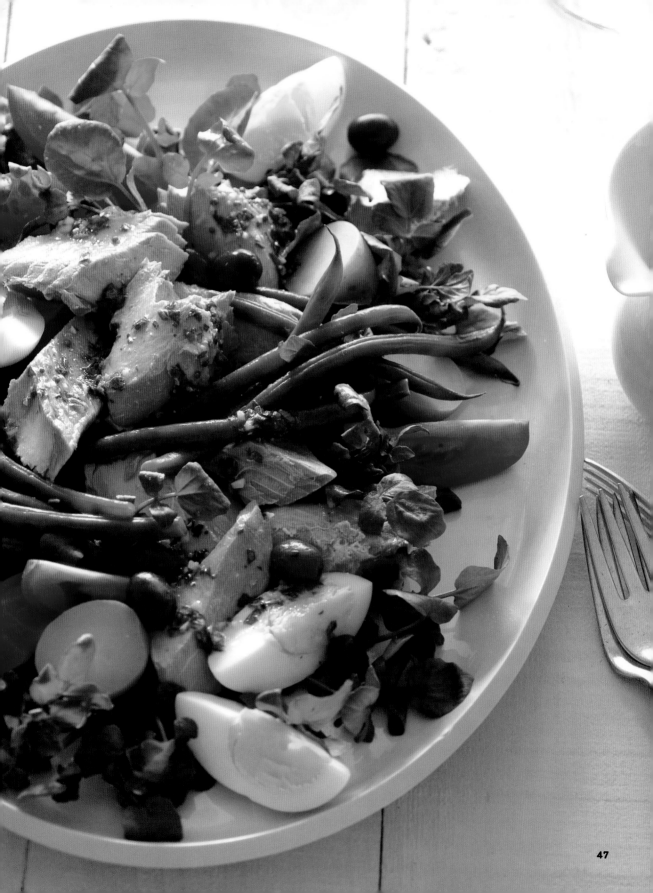

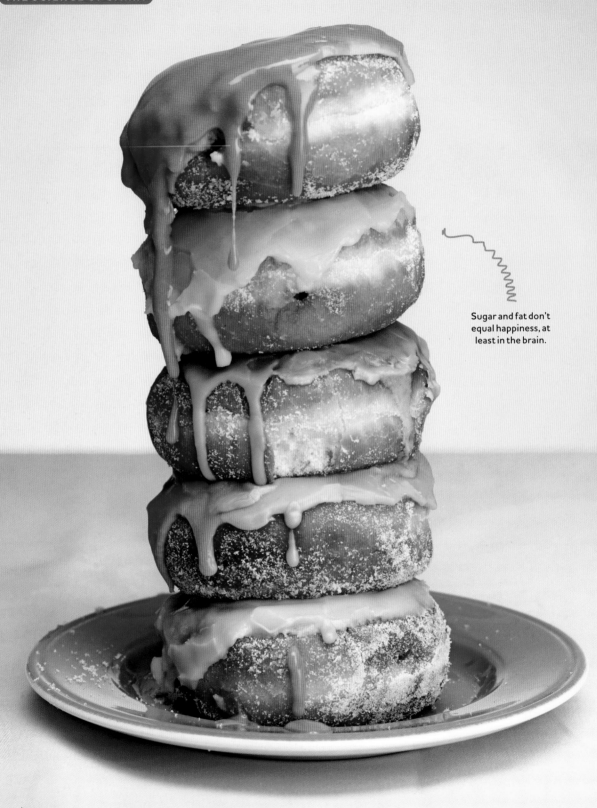

Sugar and fat don't equal happiness, at least in the brain.

The *Happiness* DIET

*

THINK THAT MEANS ALL THE SWEETS YOU CAN EAT? THINK AGAIN. HERE'S THE REAL (SCIENTIFIC) DEAL.

Food has long been linked to our emotions, at least in popular culture. We talk about comfort foods, eating our feelings, and drowning our sorrows in a pint of Häagen-Dazs. It's like we've always known intuitively that foods can affect our moods; the irony is that, in many ways, until recently we've gotten that relationship all wrong. Those kinds of so-called comfort foods are part of what has been dubbed the standard American diet, or SAD, which is typically high in refined carbs, sugar and processed foods—exactly the nutrients that may, to the contrary, be detrimental to our mental health.

The emerging field of research that combines nutrition with psychology has become so mainstream that it has its own name: nutritional psychiatry. In that field, studies have been piling up that show that societies following a more traditional diet—vegetables, fruits, nuts and whole grains, seafood plus some meats—have lower levels of mental health conditions such as depression and anxiety. And now, that connection between diet and mood disorders is being confirmed in more precise clinical studies.

PROOF IS IN THE PUDDING

One of them, aptly called the SMILES trial, was published in the journal *BMC Medicine* in 2017. A randomized, controlled clinical trial (the gold standard in research) of people diagnosed with moderate to severe depression, it found that those who were coached by a dietitian to follow a Mediterranean-style diet for 12 weeks experienced significant improvements in mood compared to people who simply received social support that did not include dietary advice. By the end of the study, around 30% of patients receiving the nutritional support were in remission for their depression, compared with only 8% of the social support group.

Another article, a meta-analysis of randomized, controlled studies published in the journal *Psychosomatic Medicine* in 2018, looked at 16 different studies and found that "dietary interventions significantly reduced depressive symptoms." It concluded that "dietary interventions hold promise as a novel intervention for reducing symptoms of depression across the population." Changing what you eat may yield surprisingly quick results, as shown in another randomized, controlled study of depressed young adults published in the journal *PLOS One* in 2019. It showed that those who followed a Mediterranean-style diet for just three weeks "had significantly lower self-reported depression symptoms than the control group" and that those changes persisted for at least three months after the study ended.

What was this magical depression-relieving diet? Participants were told to increase their intake of veggies to five servings a day and fruits to two to three a day, along with eating whole grains, proteins such as fish, meat or tofu, unsweetened dairy, nuts and seeds, and olive oil, while decreasing refined carbs, sugar, fatty or processed meats and soft drinks. "The evidence is growing

Sleep, Moods and Foods

GETTING ADEQUATE REST IS KEY NOT ONLY TO OPTIMAL BRAIN FUNCTION IN GENERAL BUT TO EMOTIONAL BALANCE. SO MAKE A MEAL, OR LATE-EVENING SNACK, OF THESE CHOICES.

Serotonin-boosting nutrients like those in vegetables and whole grains have an important role in regulating the wake-sleep cycle—and that is important to your brain's health in another way: Sleep is absolutely essential to good brain function. And foods can help to make that happen.

Numerous studies have shown an association between sleep duration and quality and cognitive function. One found that people with insufficient sleep (fewer than four hours a night) showed significant cognitive impairment over time. Sleep is when your brain repairs and rejuvenates and clears out detritus that can lead to dementia, explains neuropsychiatrist Louann Brizendine, MD. "All day, billions of neurons are firing and signaling, which produces waste byproducts, including two proteins—tau and B-amyloid— that have been linked to Alzheimer's. During sleep, neural activity quiets down, and 'garbage collector' cells called microglia can clear out the waste." Insufficient sleep short-circuits that process, allowing tau, B-amyloid and other waste products to build up and disrupt brain function. (For more on the importance of sleep, see page 128).

The Sleep Foundation recommends these foods and their key ingredients to help you get a better night's sleep:

FATTY FISH vitamin D and omega-3 fatty acids, which regulate serotonin

KIWI antioxidants and serotonin

MILK AND MALTED MILK vitamins B and D; melatonin

NUTS melatonin, magnesium and zinc

TART CHERRIES AND TART CHERRY JUICE melatonin and antioxidants

TURKEY tryptophan, a sleep-promoting amino acid

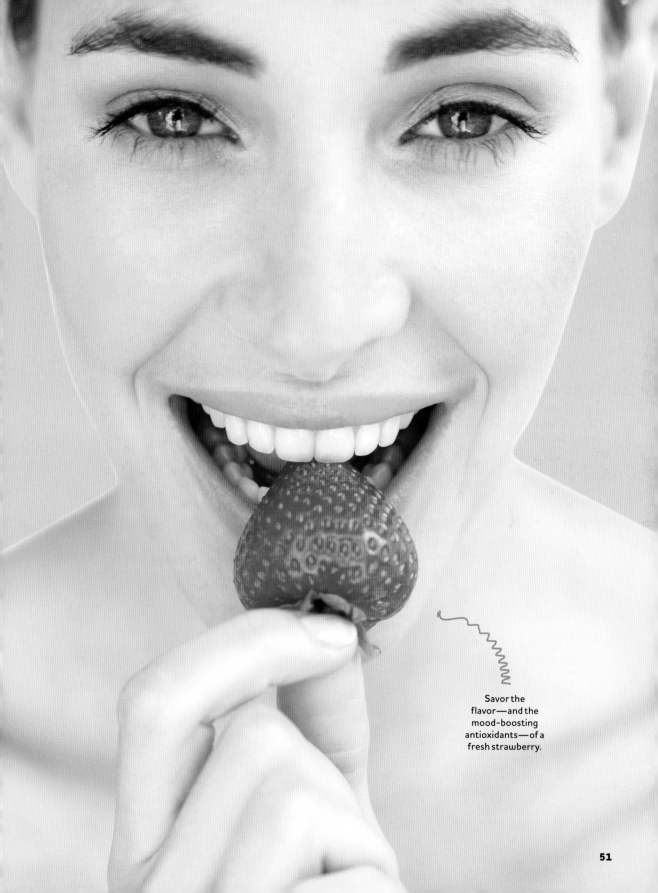

Savor the flavor—and the mood-boosting antioxidants—of a fresh strawberry.

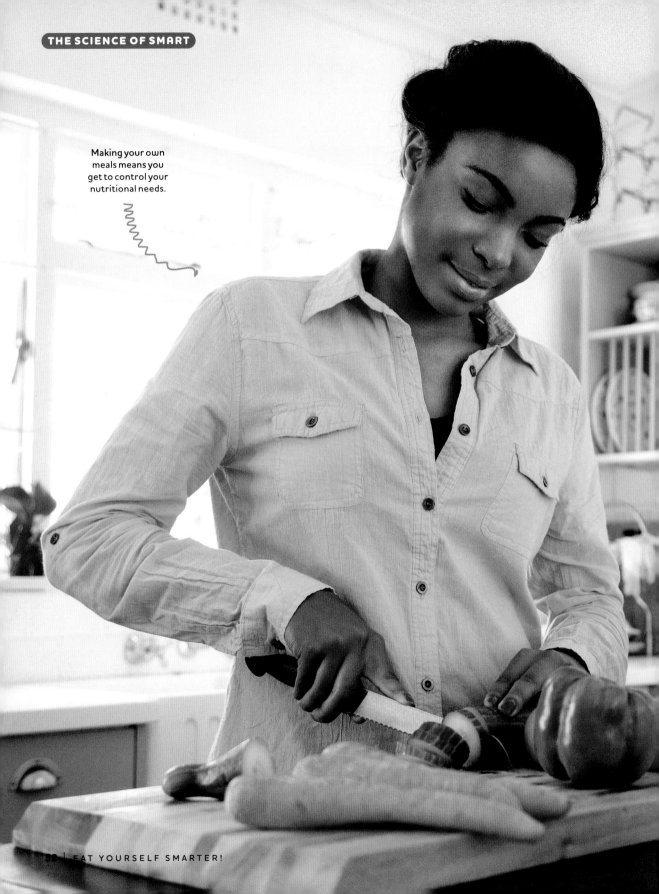

Making your own meals means you get to control your nutritional needs.

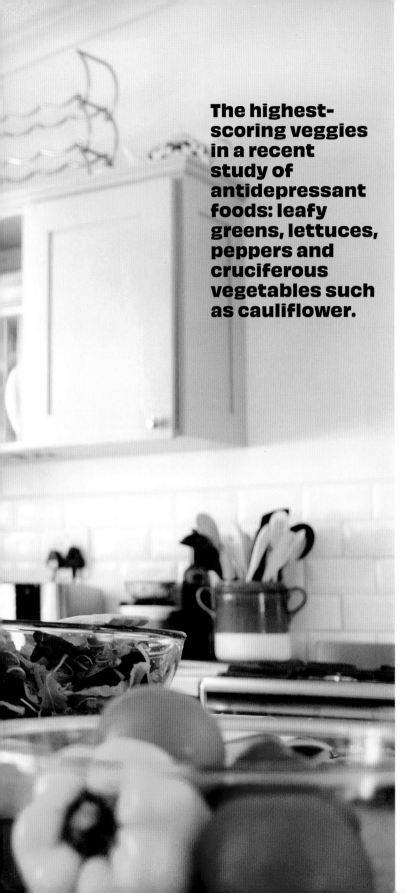

The highest-scoring veggies in a recent study of antidepressant foods: leafy greens, lettuces, peppers and cruciferous vegetables such as cauliflower.

that food choice is strongly implicated in mental health risk, and also that diet is a powerful intervention to treat depression," says the study's co-author, Laura LaChance, PhD, a lecturer in brain and therapeutics at the University of Toronto. LaChance, along with psychiatrist Drew Ramsey, MD, founder of the Brain Food Clinic in New York City, is the co-author of several studies looking at nutrition's impact on mental health.

One of these, published in the *World Journal of Psychiatry*, produced an evidence-based Antidepressant Food Score (AFS) identifying food micronutrients and whole foods that have been shown to influence mood. But what's the secret? How can the foods we eat "adjust" our brain chemistry to make us happier and less anxious? Read on.

MOOD MECHANISMS

Until recently, neurotransmitters were seen as the primary key to brain chemistry, says LaChance. These are chemical messengers with familiar names such as serotonin and dopamine, which carry signals between brain cells—and some of the most important of these involve mood, emotion and concentration. Dopamine, for instance, is known as a "pleasure or reward" neurotransmitter because it is released during pleasurable activities (and is highly tied to addictive behaviors). Serotonin plays a key role in depression and anxiety, which is why antidepressants, like Prozac, work to increase the availability of serotonin in the brain.

The brain can't manufacture these mood-related neurotransmitters without the help of various nutrients, including folate and other B vitamins, vitamins C and E and essential trace minerals such as selenium and magnesium. Tons of research shows that being deficient in these nutrients—which are plentiful in many fresh fruits and vegetables, along with certain protein-rich foods—can lead to mood disturbances.

But neurotransmitters aren't the whole story, and emerging studies, including some by LaChance and Ramsey, have been documenting other important nutritional elements of mental health. "Right now we are seeing a lot of research in the areas of inflammation, oxidative stress and the microbiome, among others," says LaChance. "For instance, elevated markers of inflammation, meaning inflammatory cytokines, have been found in the body and brains of people with depression, bipolar disorder, psychosis and other conditions. And since oxidative stress is a natural byproduct

Research in the growing field of nutritional psychiatry is finding what you eat affects how you feel—and how you behave.

of normal metabolism, and the brain has a high rate of metabolic activity, the brain tends to be exposed to higher amounts of oxidative stress compared to other tissues."

How does that translate to nutrients? Some, like omega-3 fatty acids, are powerfully anti-inflammatory, for one thing. Other foods, including most fruits and vegetables, are rich in antioxidant nutrients such as vitamin C, beta-carotene, lycopene and many polyphenols, which fight oxidative stress. As far as the gut microbiome, says LaChance, the complex carbohydrates in foods such as legumes, starchy vegetables and whole grains are high in fiber, "which act as prebiotics to support the growth of a healthy microbiome."

Bottom line: To feel not only healthier and smarter but also happier, say buh-bye to the sweets and simple carbs and hello to fresh veggies, fruits, fish and some of the other winners found in the "Top Antidepressant Foods" chart, left.

Top Antidepressant Foods

A comprehensive analysis published in the *World Journal of Psychiatry* in 2018 came up with an Antidepressant Food Score to identify foods that are the best sources of nutrients shown to play a role in the prevention of—and promotion of recovery from—depressive disorders. Consider this a cheat sheet for your Happiness Diet:

ANIMAL FOODS
* Clams and mussels
* Crab
* Liver and other organ meats
* Octopus
* Oysters

PLANT FOODS
* Fresh herbs (cilantro, basil and parsley)
* Mustard, turnip and beet greens
* Spinach
* Swiss chard
* Watercress

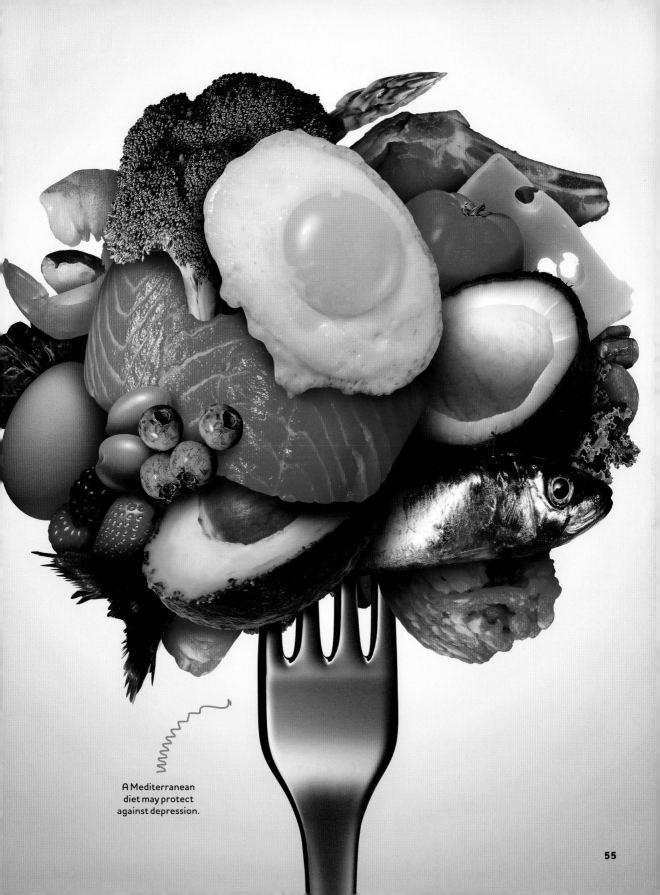

A Mediterranean diet may protect against depression.

In addition to your brain, salmon is good for the heart, skin, bones and more.

YOUR FOOD CHOICES PLAY A HUGE ROLE IN KEEPING YOUR COGNITIVE FACULTIES AGILE AND HIGH-FUNCTIONING AS YOU GET OLDER. FOLLOW THIS PRESCRIPTION, STARTING NOW, FOR AN AGE-RESISTANT BRAIN.

Staying SHARP

Anyone over "a certain age" can attest to the alarm that is triggered by losing track of your keys or forgetting someone's name. "Am I getting dementia?" is the common worry. In fact, it is the most common worry. A recent study by the Alzheimer's Association found that, among Americans age 60 and over, more were afraid of getting dementia (35%) than of having cancer (23%) or a stroke (15%). Another survey, from the University of Michigan, found that almost half of respondents over 50 thought they were likely to develop dementia in their lifetime. The bad news is that there is some reason for the anxiety.

Rates of dementia, an umbrella term covering cognitive decline (of which 70% is diagnosed as Alzheimer's, the most prevalent form), increased around the world by 117% between 1990 and 2016, according to data from the Global Burden of Diseases, Injuries, and Risk Factors Study in 2016. And in the U.S., the Alzheimer's Association documents that while deaths from heart disease between 2000 and 2018 have decreased almost 8%, deaths from Alzheimer's disease during the same period have shot up 146%.

Dementia is considered a disease of aging, so in that regard perhaps it's no surprise that it is rising along with the increase in longevity. Over the past three decades, the number of Americans age 90 and older has nearly tripled, and that age group is now the fastest-growing segment of the American population. But it's not that simple, as more and more evidence emerges that lifestyle interventions, carried out over decades of adult life, have an enormous impact on dementia risk—and chief among them are diet and exercise. A long-term study by the Rush University Medical Center in Chicago reported in 2019 that combining five habits, including eating healthier and exercising regularly, can lower the risk of developing Alzheimer's by an astounding 60%.

"So many of our lifestyle choices play a role in determining the destiny of our brains," says neurologist David Perlmutter, MD, an expert in brain function and dementia and the author of *Grain Brain* and other books. "But there is no question that our dietary choices belong at the top of the list."

Studies are showing that what you eat and how you live can lower your risk of dementia, even if you have a genetic predisposition to Alzheimer's due to the gene variant APOE-4 or other markers. A 2019 *JAMA* study found that a favorable lifestyle was associated with a lower dementia risk among participants with high genetic risk. "Our genetics actually play a minor role in determining our overall risk for dementia,"

Perlmutter explains. "Far more influential are lifestyle issues over which we have control like diet, exercise, quality and quantity of sleep and even our level of social engagement."

THE RIGHT DIET

Research is also supplying many answers to the question of which dietary habits are most protective against cognitive decline, with numerous studies pointing to the famous Mediterranean diet—high in vegetables, fruits, olive oil, whole grains, fish, nuts and seeds; lower in red meats and processed foods—as the best brain insurance as you get older. "One recent study, at the University of Illinois in people ages 65 to 75, found that those following the Mediterranean diet had improved function in the frontoparietal network in the brain," says Louann Brizendine, MD, a neuropsychiatrist and author of *The Female Brain* and *The Male Brain*. "That's the network that helps you focus on

Foods such as leafy green vegetables, berries, whole grains, fish, beans, nuts and olive oil may help reduce the risk of dementia.

tasks and follow goal-oriented behavior. The diet boosts the brain's efficiency, meaning it can communicate better across networks."

The Mediterranean diet can also help maintain the brain's size as you age, a key sign of cognitive health. For instance, a 2015 study in the journal *Neurology* examined brain volume and cortical thickness using MRIs in 674 elderly adults; both of these measures show whether the brain is aging healthfully, without shrinkage. Researchers found that adherence to a Mediterranean-type diet was associated with less brain atrophy, making their brains look about five years younger. Another study, this one published in the journal *Alzheimer's & Dementia* in 2020, evaluated almost 8,000 people and found that those who ate a Mediterranean diet had higher cognitive function and less risk of cognitive impairment. That study also found a specific link between eating fish more than twice a week and slower cognitive decline.

What's so special about the Mediterranean plan, and fish in particular? One big factor: omega-3 fatty acids, which are plentiful in both. These polyunsaturated lipids make up constituents of cell membranes and are essential for normal brain function, and numerous studies have shown that a

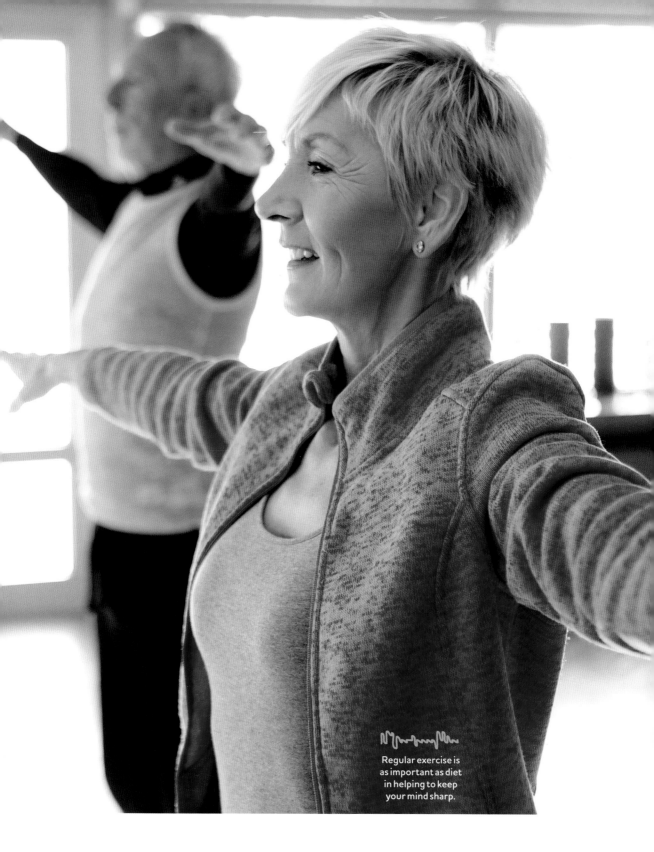

Regular exercise is
as important as diet
in helping to keep
your mind sharp.

dietary deficiency of omega-3s is associated with impaired learning, memory and dementia. The standard American diet tends to be low in omega-3s, and although researchers have tested fish-oil supplements, so far they have come up empty-handed; there is no substitute yet shown for consuming the fats in food.

The abundance of fruits and vegetables in the Mediterranean plan is also key, because such foods are rich in compounds called polyphenols. An analysis in the journal *Foods* in 2019 found that polyphenol consumption "has been reported in 23 developed countries to decrease the rates of dementia, depression and Alzheimer's disease," concluding that "polyphenols can be considered potential compounds for the treatment and prevention of cognitive impairment," leading to better connections between synapses in key brain regions.

INFLAMM-AGING

Equally important is what the Mediterranean diet *doesn't* contain, most particularly lots of red meat, processed foods and highly refined grains. All of those foods are inflammatory, and inflammation is your brain's worst enemy. The best thing you can do to protect your brain from cognitive decline and dementia, says Perlmutter, "is to reduce inflammation, and dietary choices are the most powerful

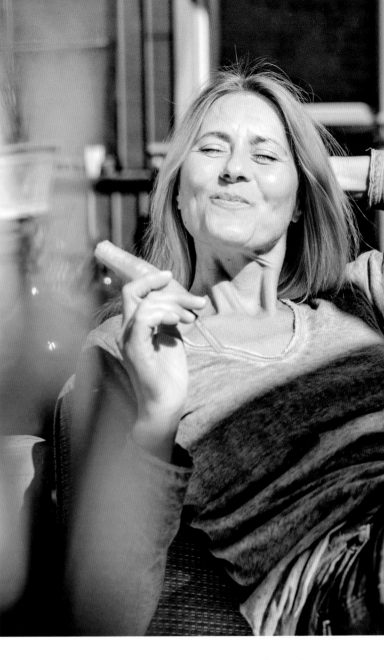

tools for this. Inflammation is central to the progressive decline in functionality and vitality of brain cells, which are hallmarks of the aging brain." The process of inflammation is so important to brain decline, says Perlmutter, that there is now a specific term

to express that relationship: "inflamm-aging."

One reason a diet high in sugar and refined carbohydrates is inflammatory is that it can lead to type 2 diabetes, which has been rising at exponential rates in the U.S. There is an intricate

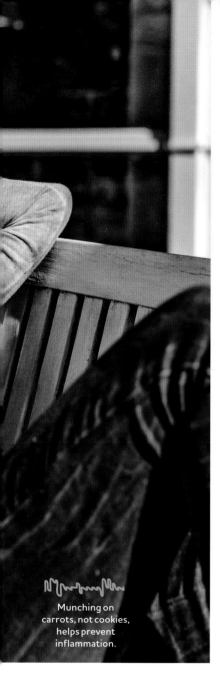

Munching on carrots, not cookies, helps prevent inflammation.

That in turn overstimulates the immune system, which sends out inflammatory molecules called cytokines that can injure the brain. "Recent research has found that diabetes greatly increases your risk of Alzheimer's, along with shrinkage of the hippocampus," says Brizendine. "That has led some researchers to call Alzheimer's 'type 3 diabetes.'"

Both diabetes and overweight are part of a cluster of conditions called metabolic syndrome (MetS), which also includes high blood pressure, high blood sugar levels and abnormal cholesterol levels. MetS, like diabetes, has soared in recent years, now affecting about one-third of American adults, and it can induce systemic inflammation. A study in the journal *Frontiers in Neuroscience* in 2018 describes how MetS can weaken the blood-brain barrier (BBB), letting in more toxins and inflammatory molecules and decreasing removal of waste products from the brain (buildup of waste products in the brain is a hallmark of Alzheimer's disease). The breakdown of the BBB, the study concludes, can lead to cognitive impairment.

The bottom line: When it comes to the long, healthy life of your brain, what you eat now makes an outsize difference to how clearly you will be thinking decades from now.

relationship between blood glucose and brain function: While glucose from the blood is the brain's favorite fuel, if you regularly take in too many carbs, you can set in motion a process that leads to high blood sugar and insulin resistance.

TOP ANTI-AGING BRAIN FOODS

REMEMBER, WHEN IT COMES TO FIGHTING DEMENTIA, WHAT YOU LEAVE OUT IS AS IMPORTANT AS WHAT YOU TAKE IN. FOLLOW THIS DO'S-AND-DON'TS GUIDE:

DO EAT
* Berries
* Cruciferous veggies (broccoli, Brussels sprouts, cauliflower)
* Fish (salmon, tuna)
* Leafy greens (kale, spinach, lettuce)
* Nuts (walnuts, almonds)

DON'T EAT
* Fast foods
* Processed meats (salami, bacon)
* Refined grains (white flour, white rice)
* Sugary drinks
* Sweets (cookies, cakes)

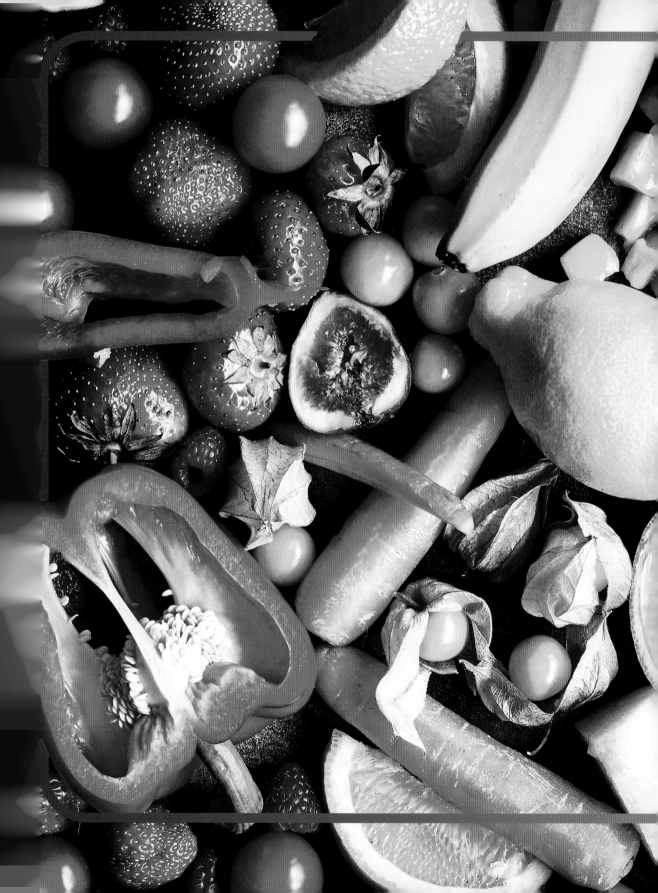

CHAPTER 2

The Power of
FOOD

MEET YOUR NEURONS' BEST FRIENDS:
THE FRUITS, VEGETABLES, PROTEINS, FATS AND
OTHER OPTIONS THAT FUEL COGNITION.

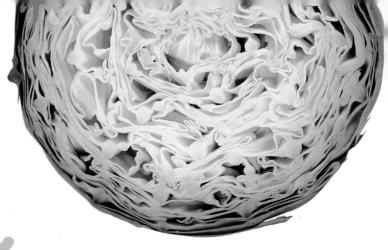

A single cup of cabbage has nearly a day's worth of brain-boosting vitamin K.

Go GREEN

* ...AND YELLOW AND ORANGE AND RED...VEGGIES ARE YOUR BRAIN'S FIRST LINE OF DEFENSE, AND THESE CHOICES ARE THE BEST OF THE BUNCH.

There's a reason this entire section leads off with vegetables: You literally cannot go wrong by eating these powerhouse plant foods. That's why mothers everywhere drill this mantra into their offspring: "Eat your vegetables!" Within the vast universe of veggies, though, some are especially rich in brain-boosting nutrients, delivering bioactive compounds that directly promote brain health and function. One critical group of these is called polyphenols, which a 2019 study in the journal *Foods* concluded have been shown by "large amounts of previous literature" to have a positive effect on "neuroprotection and antioxidant and anti-inflammatory capacity." Add to polyphenols a vast array of brain-healthy vitamins, essential fatty acids and other nutrients that are plentiful in vegetables and you have the best incentive to make them the largest food group on your plate. Look for these in particular:

BROCCOLI AND OTHER CRUCIFEROUS VEGGIES

Both the stems and the crowns of broccoli are in a category of their own when it comes to

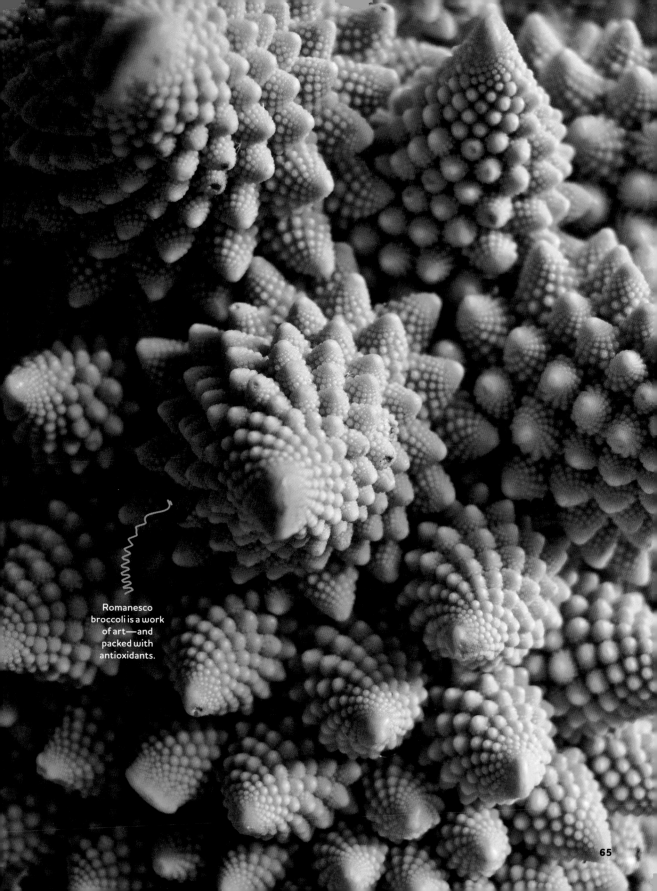

Romanesco broccoli is a work of art—and packed with antioxidants.

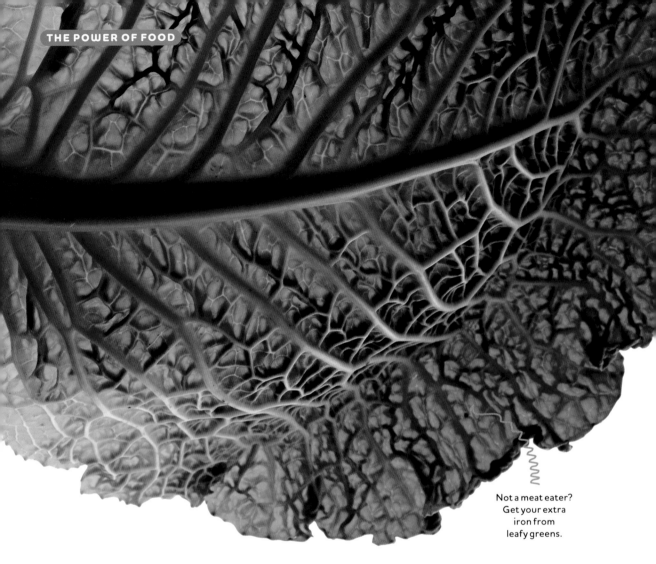

Not a meat eater? Get your extra iron from leafy greens.

brain function, while other crucifers such as Brussels sprouts and cauliflower are close runners-up. Broccoli is packed with antioxidant and anti-inflammatory compounds, which reduce damage to brain cells caused by oxidative stress, and is very high in vitamin K, delivering more than 100% of the RDI in a one-cup serving.

That fat-soluble vitamin has specific neurological benefits: It is essential for forming sphingolipids, a type of fat that's densely packed into brain cells, according to a study in *Advances in Nutrition*, and other studies have linked a higher intake of vitamin K to better memory.

Other research, published in the journal *BioMed Research International*, found that broccoli consumption affected the hippocampus—a part of the brain involved in processing the response to stressful events—by lowering levels of the stress hormone corticosterone. Since stressful events are believed to increase production of free radicals in the brain and other organs, and corticosterone itself can be damaging if it circulates for too long, reducing the stress response can be neuroprotective. Broccoli is also rich in glucosinolates, which the body breaks down into biologically active compounds called isothiocyanates; these compounds have been shown to reduce oxidative stress, potentially lowering the risk of neurodegenerative diseases.

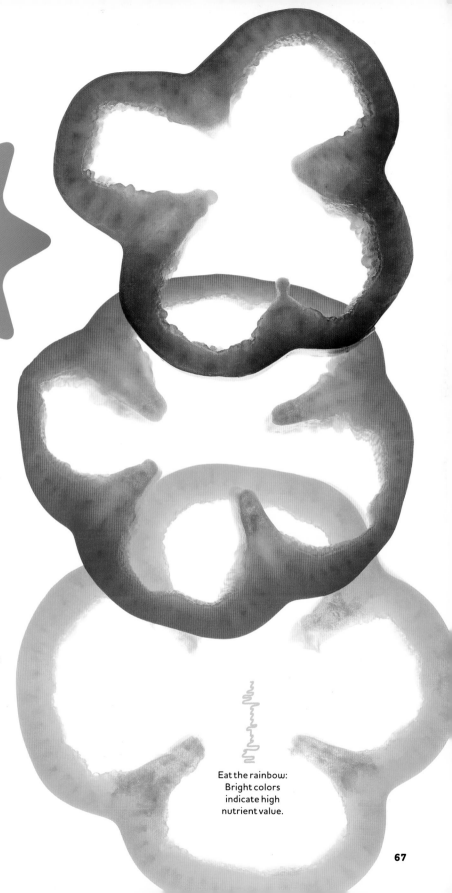

Simple Swap

INSTEAD OF
Spaghetti

EAT
Beet, carrot or zucchini noodles
(Buy a spiralizer, or purchase
prepped veggie "zoodles" at the
supermarket. Cook in a little
water until desired softness;
strain and season or sauce.)

COOK IT These veggies are
super versatile; you can steam or
roast them as a side, puree them
into a soup, cook them into egg
dishes such as souffles or quiches
or toss into pastas and stir-fries.
Cauliflower can be "riced" or
mashed as a sub for potatoes.

LEAFY GREENS

This group—which includes
spinach, Swiss chard, kale,
collard greens and arugula,
among others—tops the charts
for all aspects of health,
including disease prevention, but
its brain-protective ingredients
are particularly potent. Many
of these greens are high in iron,
which has been shown to help
normalize cognitive function;
vitamin K; vitamin E, which
protects neurons from oxidative
stress in the brain and nervous
system and has been shown to

Eat the rainbow:
Bright colors
indicate high
nutrient value.

reduce cognitive decline in the elderly; and folate, which is so key to brain health throughout life that it is essential both to neural development in the fetus and to preventing or slowing memory loss in the aging.

COOK IT Most often, greens come to the table either steamed or sauteed as a side, or raw as a base for salads. Expand your repertoire by cooking and chopping them as an ingredient in tarts, quiches and omelets; tossing into soups and pastas; or topping with cheese for a gratin.

ORANGE ROOTS AND SQUASH

"Orange" is the operative word here, because it's a signifier of the presence of beta-carotene, a powerful antioxidant that,

Want a sharper memory? Skip the expensive pills and load up on these beta-carotene-filled capsules of goodness.

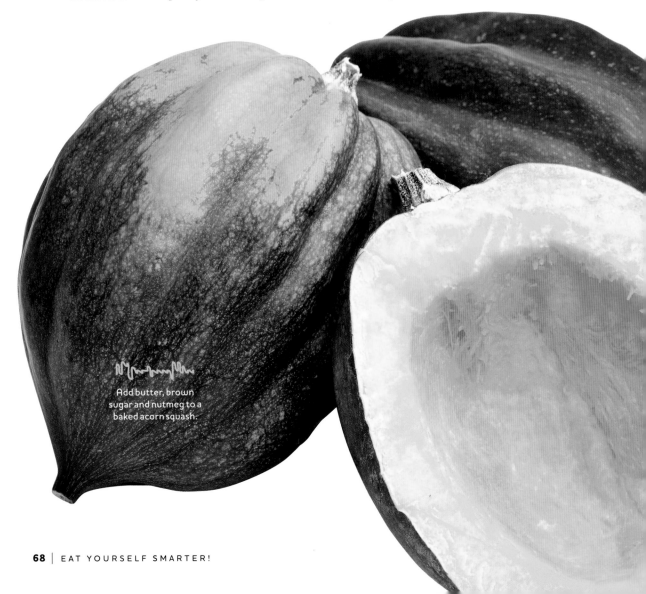

Add butter, brown sugar and nutmeg to a baked acorn squash.

like the phytochemicals in leafy greens, has myriad preventative health benefits—but especially for the brain. A 2019 study in the journal *Biomolecules* linked beta-carotene to improvement in cognitive function in mice, joining many other studies suggesting a beneficial impact of the antioxidant on the memory-regulating parts of the brain, such as the amygdala and hippocampus.

These groups of vegetables include nutrient-dense roots such as sweet potatoes, carrots and beets (which are admittedly more red than orange, but equally packed with nutrients); and winter squash such as butternut, acorn and delicata. Most of them are rich not only in beta-carotene but in other brain-boosting compounds like anthocyanins, a potent type of polyphenol, and vitamin A.

COOK IT Squash and root vegetables are delicious roasted, whether whole (as with a baked sweet potato) or cut up. Sprinkle them with a little salt to bring out their natural sweetness. Their relatively high sugar content will produce a sweet-and-savory, caramelized result. These also cook down well into a pureed soup that is the essence of vitamin-filled healthfulness.

Special Mentions

IN ADDITION TO THE GROUPS OF VEGGIES DESCRIBED HERE, SOME EXIST IN A CLASS OF THEIR OWN. THEY'RE SO FULL OF COGNITION-BOOSTING NUTRIENTS THAT YOU SHOULD PUT THEM ON THE MENU AS OFTEN AS POSSIBLE. LOOK FOR THESE SUPERFOODS:

ASPARAGUS Loaded to the gills with folate, these stalks are also rich in vitamin E, anti-inflammatory compounds and fiber to feed your "second brain," aka your all-important microbiome.

BELL PEPPERS Antioxidants, including beta-carotene and vitamin C, are these sweet veggies' calling card, helping to reduce neuron-damaging inflammation in the brain.

MUSHROOMS The health benefits of these magical fungi are many—including lowering the risk of hypertension, inflammation and liver disease—but they also have specific cognitive effects, according to recent research. In addition to boasting antioxidant and anti-inflammatory properties, mushrooms are also one of the richest sources of a compound called ergothioneine, which may help explain studies that show mushroom consumption may boost the brain's processing speed and reduce the risk of cognitive impairment.

TURMERIC ROOT Most people think of turmeric as a powder or a supplement, but in its natural form, it is a root with a powerful bioactive compound called curcumin. Researchers keep finding new benefits to curcumin, including that it has been shown to cross the blood-brain barrier and directly enter the brain, boosting brain-derived neurotrophic factor (BDNF), a type of growth hormone that helps brain cells grow. It's also a potent antioxidant and anti-inflammatory that has been linked to improved memory and higher levels of serotonin and dopamine, both of which improve mood.

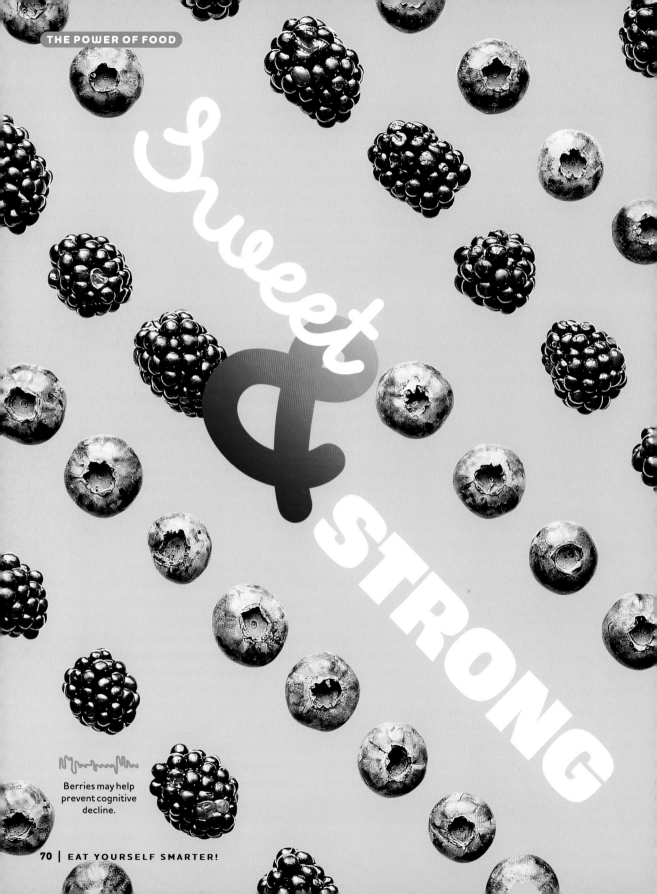

Sweet & STRONG

Berries may help prevent cognitive decline.

✱ SWAP A BAG OF CANDY FOR A HANDFUL OF BERRIES, MANGO SLICES, OR A WHOLE ORANGE. YOUR BRAIN WILL THANK YOU FOR THE BOOST (AND THE TASTE!).

Fruits have caught some nutritional shade in the past few years, as concern about dietary sugar intake has grown. After all, these gems were created by nature to be super-attractive, i.e. sweet, to the palates of the animal kingdom. The reason for this is pure reproductive Darwinism: Botanically, a fruit is a mature ovary of the plant, and each of the seeds it harbors contains an embryo plant. The more a plant's fruits can entice animals to eat them, the further those seeds will be spread, ensuring the "birth" of ever more plants and the survival of the species. Enter juicy berries and luscious grapes.

And also enter the good news: The sugars in fruit, naturally occurring and delivered in a package together with rich nutrients and fiber, acts very differently in the body than highly processed sugar packaged into soft drinks, white bread and sweets. First of all, fruits have much less sugar than processed foods, and the sugar it does contain is more complex. Its breakdown in the bloodstream is slowed by the abundant fiber in fruits, so you don't get on the blood-glucose roller coaster of simple sugars that can lead to systemic inflammation and diseases like type 2 diabetes.

Beyond that, though, is the pure power of fruits' phytochemicals—the reason why many varieties qualify as true brain foods. In addition to numerous antioxidants and anti-inflammatories, most fruits contain copious amounts of bioactive molecules called flavonoids. Studies have shown that flavonoids help regulate cellular activity, lower inflammation and fight off free radicals that cause oxidative stress, especially in the brain. According to a study in the journal *Neural Regeneration Research*, some fruit-based flavonoids called anthocyanins have been found to accumulate in the brain and help improve communication between brain cells. Another study, in the *Journal of Agricultural and Food Chemistry*, found that adding anthocyanin-rich blueberries to the diets of older adults improved memory and may delay age-related short-term memory loss.

An apple (eat the skin) brings fiber and antioxidants with it.

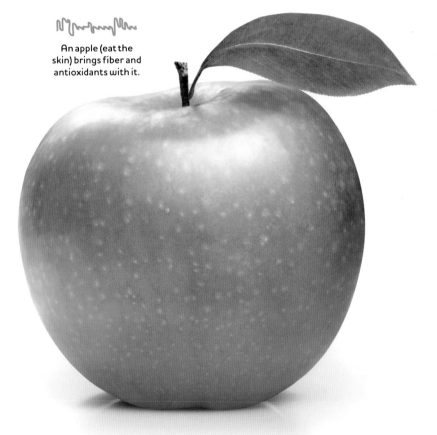

The actions of flavonoids in the brain are multifaceted, working through several different mechanisms to boost brain function. One involves blood flow, according to a study in the journal *Foods*. That study found that flavonoids can increase cerebral blood flow, which in turn improves synaptic plasticity—the ability of the brain's synapses, the junction between nerve cells, to communicate with each other. The better that communication is, the clearer your thoughts, learning and memory. Other research,

reported in the *British Journal of Nutrition*, suggests that flavonoids may influence the underlying cellular architecture in the brain, protecting neurons and enhancing their function. The result: quicker cognition and more effective memory storage. All fruits are good, but for the most benefits, seek out the following varieties in particular.

BERRIES

These red, blue and black bite-size jewels are the royalty of the fruit realm—at least when it comes to brain function—and blueberries top the hierarchy. They are particularly rich in anthocyanins, as well as other

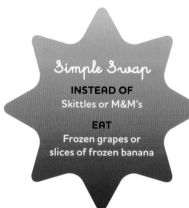

Simple Swap
INSTEAD OF
Skittles or M&M's
EAT
Frozen grapes or slices of frozen banana

plant compounds with anti-inflammatory and antioxidant effects, which reduce any collateral damage to the brain from oxidative stress. Blueberries' cognitive effects can be so powerful that in one study, researchers gave a group of older adults with early memory changes wild blueberry juice daily for 12 weeks and found improvements in their memory performance on tests. Don't neglect other berries though, as choices including cranberries, raspberries, strawberries and blackberries are also rich in anthocyanins.

EAT THEM It's easy to up your intake of berries on a daily basis. Toss them on your morning oatmeal or yogurt; puree them into a smoothie; bake them into a whole-grain muffin or fruit crumble; cook them down into a compote; or just snack on them by the handful.

CITRUS FRUITS

Oranges, grapefruit, lemons and limes aren't just replete with health-promoting vitamin C; they are also rich sources of

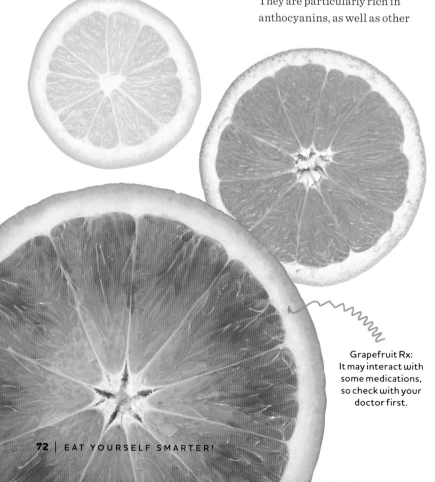

Grapefruit Rx: It may interact with some medications, so check with your doctor first.

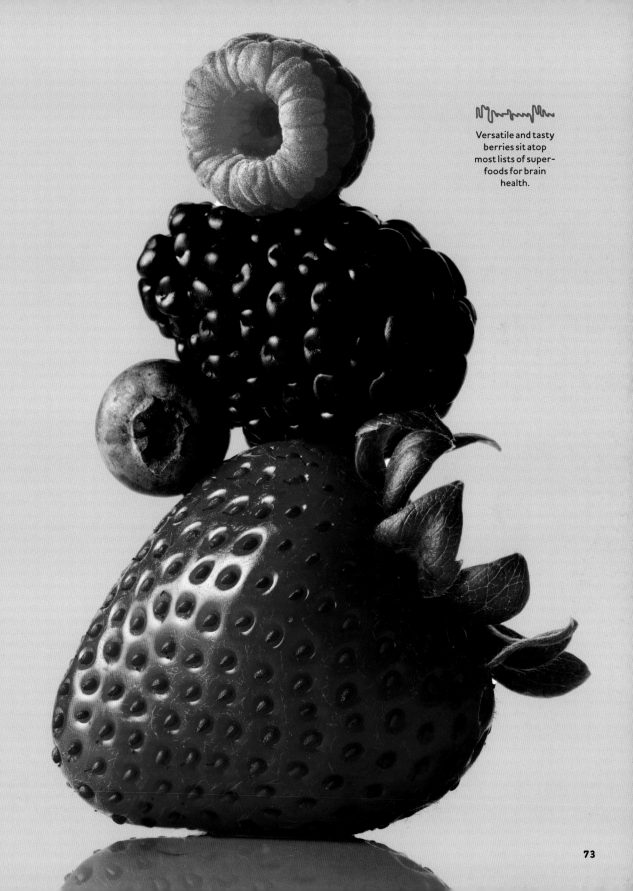

Versatile and tasty berries sit atop most lists of super-foods for brain health.

Top Picks

CERTAIN FRUITS—INCLUDING A FEW YOU MIGHT THINK OF AS VEGETABLES—ARE IN A CATEGORY OF THEIR OWN FOR THEIR ARRAY OF BRAIN BENEFITS. INCLUDE THESE IN YOUR DIET REGULARLY:

AVOCADO Often mistaken for a green veggie, this standout is botanically a large berry with a single seed (who knew?). With more potassium than bananas, numerous heart- and brain-healthy fats and loads of fiber, avocados also contain significant amounts of lutein, which is linked to better cognition. A 2017 study in the journal *Nutrients* found that people who ate one avocado a day showed a 25% increase in lutein blood levels—and improvement in their memory and problem-solving skills.

CHOCOLATE It doesn't sound like a fruit, but cocoa powder and chocolate are made from the seeds of the fruit of the cacao tree, and a study in *Chemistry Central Journal* called cacao seeds a "super fruit," citing their high levels of antioxidants, polyphenols, and flavanols—all of which aid brain health and may enhance memory. Look for dark, low-sugar chocolates with a high cacao level.

POMEGRANATE The seeds and juice of this red fruit are powerful protectors against damage from free radicals in the brain. That may reduce dementia risk: A study in *Oncotarget* found a pomegranate-rich diet had positive impacts on the brain health of mice with Alzheimer's disease, as well as other neuroprotective effects.

TOMATOES This popular fruit shares two attributes of avocados: It's often thought of as a vegetable, and it's full of brain-boosting lutein. A study in *Frontiers in Aging Neuroscience* found significant links between blood levels of lutein and cognitive health, including temporal cortex structure and "crystallized intelligence" on IQ tests.

flavonoids that have a direct effect on the brain. Some of these have anti-inflammatory effects that protect against nervous-system deterioration; other types of flavonoids in citrus, including hesperidin and apigenin, have been shown to protect brain cells and improve brain function in mice and test-tube studies. A 2016 study in the *European Journal of Nutrition* found an association between consumption of orange juice and "acute improvements in cognitive function" in healthy middle-aged males, and another, in the *British Journal of Nutrition,* found a "pronounced" association between citrus fruit consumption and cognitive performance in older adults.

EAT THEM One benefit to citrus fruits: They're very easy to transport. Toss one in your bag or briefcase daily and

A study in the *Annals of the New York Academy of Sciences* found that polyphenols contained in fruit may alter communication between neurons.

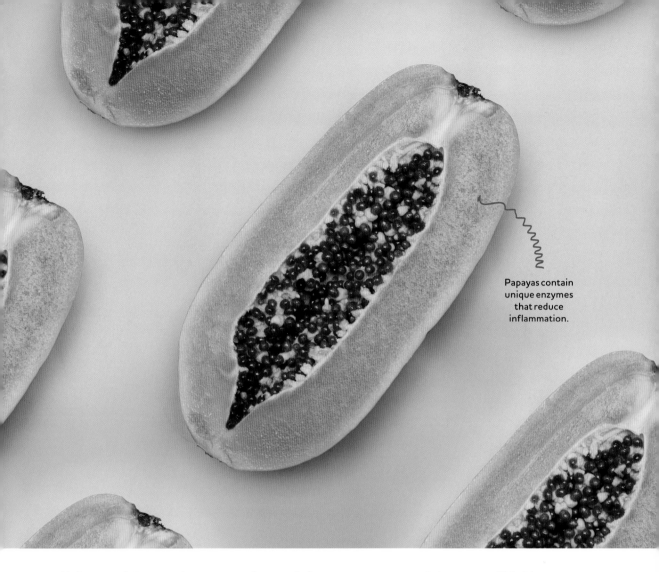

Papayas contain unique enzymes that reduce inflammation.

peel it for a snack. You can also make grapefruit a regular part of breakfast; add lemon or lime slices to your ice water or tea; serve lemon-based sauces on fish and vegetables, or add lime juice to salsas.

TROPICAL FRUITS

This category includes both the uber-familiar (bananas) and the exotic (goji berries). Most tropical fruits are packed with antioxidants that fight oxidative damage to brain cells. Some standouts include: mangoes, replete with vitamin B6 and other B vitamins that are crucial for maintaining the function of brain neurotransmitters; açai, with antioxidants that could protect against Alzheimer's, according to a study in *Neuroscience Letters*; bananas, full of magnesium (key to relaying signals between the brain and body) and potassium (which helps send more oxygen to the brain); goji berries, which studies show can increase focus and alertness; and kiwi (an excellent source of folate, which aids in cognitive development and helps repair DNA).

EAT THEM Mangoes are excellent simply peeled and sliced, or made into a sweet-and-spicy salsa. Kiwis shine in smoothie bowls or as a topping for yogurt; bananas add creaminess to smoothies or fruit salad; whirl açai or goji berries into smoothies for a tart flavor, or add them to trail mix.

KERNELS of *Truth*

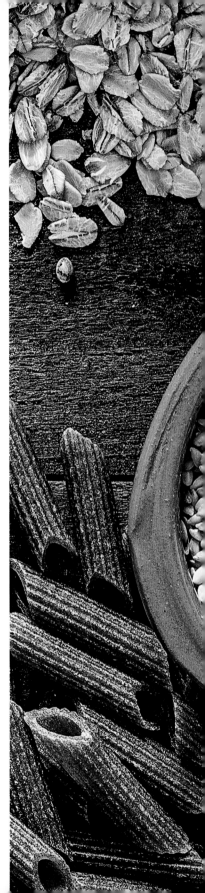

* **THE WHOLE-GRAIN STORY HAS BEEN REWRITTEN SEVERAL TIMES OVER THE PAST FEW DECADES. HERE'S THE LATEST SCIENCE ON HOW IT IMPACTS YOUR BRAIN FUNCTION.**

If you're confused about grains, you're not alone. Public opinion—and public-health advice—about their effect on human health has whipsawed back and forth for years. The 1992 Food Pyramid, issued by the United States Department of Agriculture (USDA), put the group including "bread, cereal, rice and pasta" squarely at the base of the suggested food guidelines, making it the largest category and calling for a lavish six to 11 servings a day. In contrast, "fats, oils and sweets" were relegated to a tiny triangle at the top of the pyramid, with the advice to "use sparingly."

These widely disseminated recommendations created a new market for low-fat (and nonfat) foods, especially grain-based items. (Remember Snackwell's devil's food cookies, which supermarkets couldn't even keep in stock?) But when millions of Americans turned their backs on fats and embraced grains, the result was the fastest-ever rise in obesity and an explosion in the rate of type 2 diabetes. Both of those conditions are inflammatory and linked with a higher risk of cognitive decline.

After a decade or so of that bad news, the pendulum swung again as people signed on to the Atkins and keto diets that emphasized high fat and almost no carbs—and especially, zero grains. At the same time, gluten

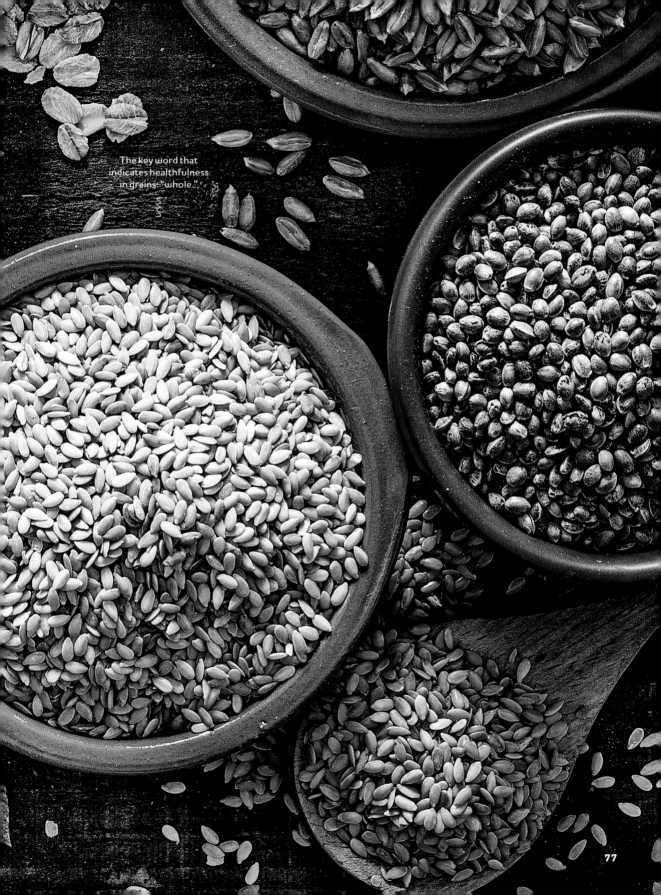

The key word that indicates healthfulness in grains: "whole."

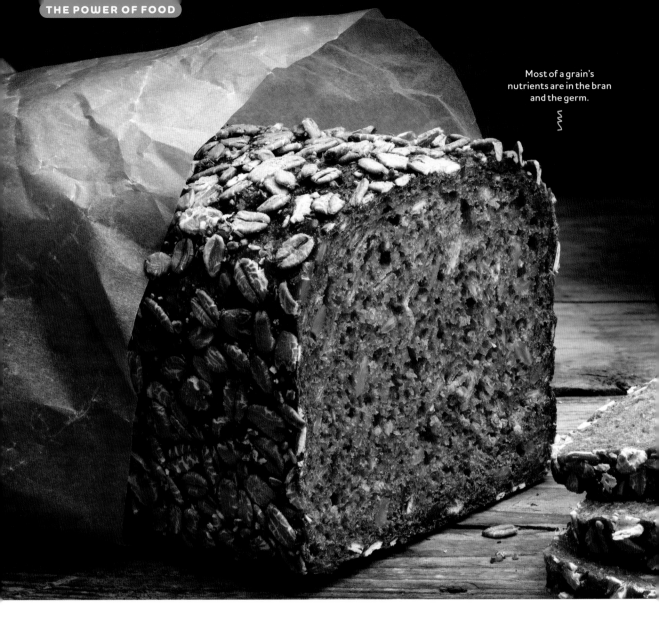

Most of a grain's nutrients are in the bran and the germ.

(a protein in wheat) emerged as the latest demon ingredient, spurring another new market, this one of "gluten-free" goods. As with all popular nutritional advice, however, the healthiest answer lies somewhere between extremes—and, in particular, with the choice of whole foods over refined and processed ones.

ESSENTIAL NUTRIENTS

There's a reason that whole grains are always mentioned as part of the healthy Mediterranean diet: They are a good source of fiber, along with many important nutrients. These include brain-friendly vitamins such as B and E, antioxidants,

minerals such as zinc and magnesium and healthy fats. Numerous studies have shown links between whole-grain intake and cognitive health, including the Women's Health Study and a 2019 study in the *American Journal of Clinical Nutrition*. The latter followed more than 500 people from young adulthood through midlife and found that those who reported consuming the most whole grains had the highest cognitive function scores.

The fiber in whole grains may play an important role in these cognitive benefits. It is linked to lower blood pressure, and anything that's good for your heart is good for your brain; it also supports beneficial bacteria in the microbiome, called the "second brain," which communicates with your "first brain" through the vagus nerve. Fiber also slows the rate at which nutrients are absorbed in the body, which helps keep blood sugar levels steady, avoiding the glucose roller-coaster effect that can lead to insulin resistance and inflammation.

Why the emphasis on "whole" grains? Because they contain the entire seed, or kernel, of the plant, including the parts that have the most nutrients. The bran, or outer skin of the seed, contains antioxidants, B vitamins and fiber. The germ, which is the embryo of the seed (like the yolk of an egg), is also rich in B vitamins, along with protein, minerals and fats. The rest of the grain, called the endosperm, mostly contains starch—explaining why the "whole" part is so key.

MODERN GRAINS

If you've heard about the Paleo diet, you know it's based on the idea that certain foods, including grains, are fairly recent additions to the human diet, due to the rise of agriculture. But in fact, studies show that millions of years ago, early humans *did* eat grains—just like they ate anything edible they could find. But they ate the entire wheat or rye seed, with all its nutrients intact. What

agriculture changed, ultimately, was both the availability of grain-based foods and their form: ground-up, refined and featuring mostly the endosperm.

Once you do that, grains become an entirely different food. First, they are denuded of almost all of their neuron-nourishing nutrients, including fiber. According to the Whole Grains Council, "Refining a grain removes about a quarter of

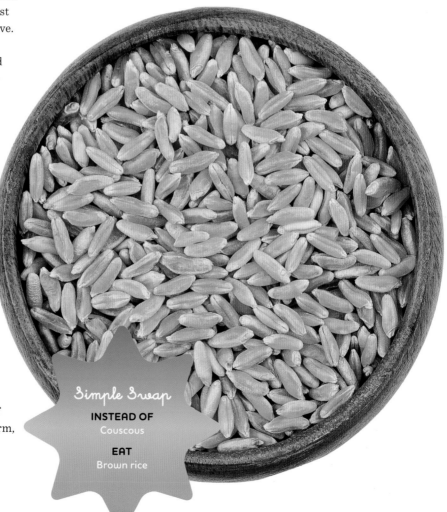

Simple Swap

INSTEAD OF
Couscous

EAT
Brown rice

the protein in a grain, and half to two-thirds or more of a score of nutrients, leaving the grain a mere shadow of its original self." But even worse for brain function, processed grains that are mostly starch break down into glucose almost immediately in the body. "By far the biggest issue of concern with respect to a diet rich in refined grains is the exposure to processed carbohydrate," says David Perlmutter, MD, an expert in brain function and dementia and author of *Grain Brain* and other books. "This ultimately opens the door to elevated blood sugar and its association with Alzheimer's disease."

Many of the grain-based foods so popular in the U.S.—breakfast cereals, breads, bagels, pizza dough, white rice—essentially act like pure sugar in the body, and sugar is highly inflammatory. Even foods marketed as "healthy," items such as granola or whole-wheat bread (much of which has almost as much white flour as whole-wheat flour), can spike blood sugar and spark inflammation.

Then there is the gluten issue. Perlmutter calls it "the sticky protein"; the word itself is Latin for "glue," because this naturally occurring protein holds products like bread together. A small proportion of the population has celiac disease, an extreme sensitivity to gluten that causes all kinds

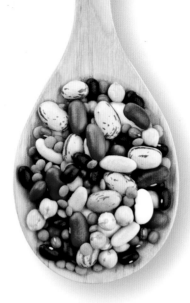

Beans have a similar mouth-feel to grains, but bring extra protein— without the gluten. Toss them in!

of symptoms. But Perlmutter and others believe that a much larger number of people have a lesser form of gluten sensitivity, an over-response of the immune system that may be causing silent damage, especially to brain function, in the form of inflammation—even in the absence of symptoms. Over the past two decades, research has emerged tying gluten to neurological issues, including a 2009 article in the journal *Medical Hypotheses* that concluded: "Gluten is linked to neurological harm in patients, both with and without evidence of celiac disease."

ANCIENT WISDOM

How to harness the goodness in grains, without the bad? One solution is to consume them the way our ancestors did: in their whole form. The current problem with foods like bread is not simply that they're very refined, but also that the wheat being grown today has been bio-engineered and hybridized in ways that may make its gluten harder for the human body to tolerate, according to Perlmutter. So consider trying some of the so-called ancient grains recently enjoying popularity, which are relatively unchanged from their original structure; some also happen to be gluten-free. "Gluten-free grains are absolutely acceptable additions to a brain-healthy diet, provided they are not refined and serving sizes are reasonable," says Perlmutter.

Gluten-free grains include brown rice, steel-cut oats, amaranth, buckwheat (gluten-free, despite the name), millet, quinoa, fonio, sorghum and teff—all loaded with vitamins, minerals and antioxidants. Certain ancient grains that do contain gluten—including kamut, spelt, freekeh and farro—have sky-high levels of nutrients and antioxidants, including carotenoids and phytosterols. Another alternative: Satisfy a yen for starch with beans, which share many of the nutrients of whole grains, minus the downsides of refining or gluten.

The Bounty of Beans

CRAVING STARCHES? TRY SOME OF THESE NUTRIENT-PACKED LEGUMES AND BEANS.

It's been proven time and again that beans and legumes, a staple of the Mediterranean diet, are brain superstars. Numerous studies have shown their benefits, including one in the *Journal of Translational Medicine* in 2017, which found that a higher consumption of legumes (more than three servings per week) in the elderly is independently associated with higher cognitive scores. And conversely, other studies have linked a lower intake of vegetables and legumes with cognitive decline. Try incorporating some of these into your soups, casseroles, dips and chilis. You'll be getting loads of fiber and these nutrients:

BLACK BEANS contain protein, folate, manganese, magnesium, thiamine, iron

CHICKPEAS contain protein, folate, manganese, iron

KIDNEY BEANS contain protein, folate, thiamine, copper, iron

LENTILS contain protein, folate, thiamine

NAVY BEANS contain protein, folate, manganese, thiamine, magnesium, iron

PEANUTS contain manganese, niacin, magnesium, folate, vitamin E, thiamine

PEAS contain folate, vitamin K, thiamine

SOYBEANS contain protein, manganese, iron, phosphorus, vitamin K, riboflavin, isoflavones

Small

Peanuts are plentiful in healthy fats, protein and fiber.

WONDERS

* THESE TINY POWERHOUSES
PROVIDE LONG-LASTING FUEL
FOR COGNITIVE HEALTH.

The most important anatomical point about seeds is this: They are essentially a plant's embryo, containing everything needed to begin life. And like eggs, another embryonic foodstuff, they are extraordinarily nutritious brain food. In common usage, most people think of nuts and seeds as two distinct types of food, but in fact they are both classified as seeds. That hard case around an edible walnut, for instance, is botanically a fruit, making the nut inside a jumbo seed.

Why is this important? The reason is something our human ancestors discovered thousands of years ago: If you put seeds in the ground and tend them, they will sprout into plants, which are great for sustaining life. But beyond that usefulness, seeds themselves supply a bonanza of life-giving nutrients when eaten as is. A recent study published in the *Proceedings of the National Academy of Sciences* found that, almost 2 million years before the development of agriculture, our forebears feasted on nuts and seeds they foraged from wild plants. Then when humans started cultivating crops about 10,000 years ago, they harvested seeds not just for planting but for eating. Flaxseed fields dotted Babylon in 3000 B.C.; in pre-Columbian America, pumpkin seeds were prized for their ability to fuel hunters seeking game. Caraway seeds became so ubiquitous in Nordic culture that they were used to flavor aquavit, the spirit that takes its name from the Latin "water of life." Seed-based dishes have been central to cooking in cultures around the world, from sesame tahini in the Middle East to cumin-laced Indian curries.

The brain-boosting nutrients in nuts and seeds include healthy fats such as omega-3 fatty acids, zinc, vitamin E, selenium, magnesium, and numerous antioxidants. To reap their benefits, expand your culinary universe by not only snacking on them plain or sprinkling them onto dishes, but also by using ground nuts and seeds in recipes and consuming nut and seed butters. Shop for these top choices:

NUTS

WALNUTS

The Harvard T.H. Chan School of Public Health puts these nuts at the top of their list for brain health, in part due to their high level of a type of omega-3 fatty acid called alpha-linolenic acid (ALA), which helps lower blood pressure and protects arteries (which in turn helps keep the brain nourished by oxygen-rich blood). A study in the *Journal of Nutrition, Health and Aging* in 2015 showed that eating walnuts may improve performance on cognitive function tests, including those for memory, concentration and information-processing speed.

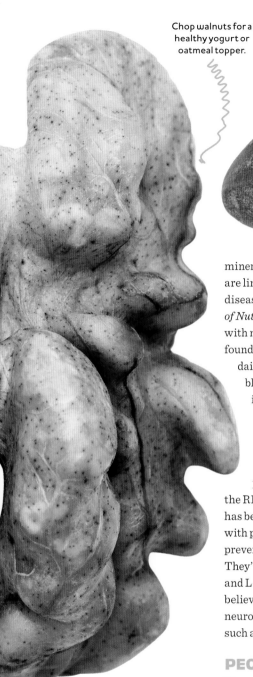

Chop walnuts for a healthy yogurt or oatmeal topper.

mineral. Low selenium levels are linked to neurodegenerative diseases, and a *European Journal of Nutrition* study in older adults with mild cognitive impairment found that eating one Brazil nut daily for six months raised blood selenium levels and improved verbal fluency and mental function.

ALMONDS

A one-quarter cup serving packs in nearly 50% of the RDA of vitamin E, which has been strongly associated with preserving memory and preventing cognitive decline. They're also rich in riboflavin and L-carnitine, which are believed to help ward off neurodegenerative diseases such as Alzheimer's.

PECANS

These have the highest level of Alzheimer's-fighting antioxidants of all edible nuts, along with plentiful monounsaturated fats, such as oleic acids, which reduce the risk of heart disease. A healthy dose of B vitamins adds to the benefits.

BRAZIL NUTS

These jumbo nuts contain ellagic acid, a type of polyphenol that has both antioxidant and anti-inflammatory properties, as well as selenium, a key antioxidant

Simple Swap
INSTEAD OF
Chips or pretzels

EAT
A handful of walnuts, pecans or almonds

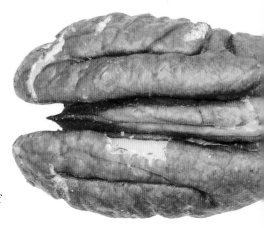

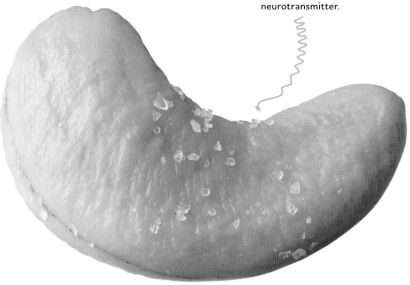

Cashews may raise levels of serotonin, a mood-boosting neurotransmitter.

SEEDS

SUNFLOWER SEEDS

These popular seeds are high in the antioxidant vitamin E, which protects brain cells from oxidative stress caused by free radicals; a 2014 review in *The Journal of Nutrition, Health, and Aging* found that vitamin E may also contribute to improved cognition and reduced risk of Alzheimer's disease.

Many of the benefits—and much of the flavor—of nuts and seeds come from their brain-boosting healthy fats, like omega-3s and oleic acids.

CASHEWS

Rich and flavorful, cashews are an excellent source of copper, which a study in the *Proceedings of the National Academy of Sciences* describes as playing "an essential role in the health of the human brain." Improper copper oxidation has been linked to several neurological disorders, including Alzheimer's and Parkinson's.

PEANUTS

Technically a legume, peanuts get an honorable mention in the nut category because of their many brain (and heart) benefits. They contain generous amounts of resveratrol, a bioactive compound found to improve blood flow to the brain in a 2016 study, as well as niacin and vitamin E, which have been shown to protect against Alzheimer's and age-related cognitive decline.

SESAME SEEDS

One of the most popular and versatile varieties of seeds, they're an excellent source of the amino acid tyrosine, which is used to produce dopamine, a neurotransmitter that helps keep the brain alert and memory sharp. The seeds also are rich in memory-boosting zinc, magnesium and vitamin B6.

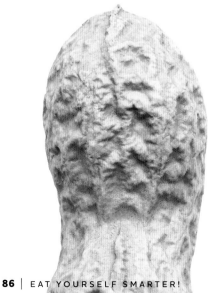

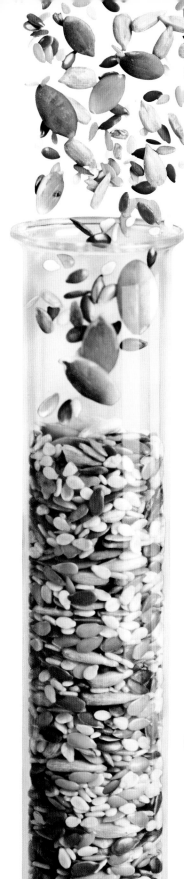

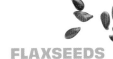

Mix and match nuts and seeds to get the most benefits.

CHIA SEEDS

Packed with fiber to feed your microbiome, as well as a surprising amount of protein, gram for gram, chia seeds contain more omega-3 fatty acids than salmon. They also have anti-inflammatory properties; one three-month study in people with diabetes, which is an inflammatory disease, showed that eating chia seeds daily reduced the level of a key marker of inflammation by 40%, while a control group who consumed wheat bran showed no significant benefit.

PUMPKIN SEEDS

A study in *Food Chemistry* found your jack-o'-lantern's leftovers contain brain-protective antioxidants. The seeds are also a good source of zinc (crucial for nerve signaling), magnesium (essential for learning and memory), copper and iron.

FLAXSEEDS

Famous for their high levels of omega-3 fatty acids, especially cardio-boosting alpha-linolenic acid (ALA), flaxseeds also fight inflammation, which damages brain neurons. A 2019 study in *Nutrients* found that baby rats given milled flaxseed or flaxseed oil had higher brain mass, suggesting better brain development. (Tip: The benefits are more available when they're ground, so toss into a smoothie.)

HEMPSEEDS

High in brain-powering magnesium, potassium and vitamin E, hempseeds were also found in a study in *Food Chemistry* to have antioxidant effects, perhaps due to their cannabidiol (CBD) content. A 2018 review in *Surgical Neurology International* suggested that because of CBD's neuroprotective and anti-inflammatory properties, the seeds (and their oil) may help with neurological conditions such as Parkinson's and Alzheimer's.

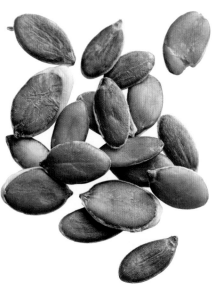

Liquid GOLD

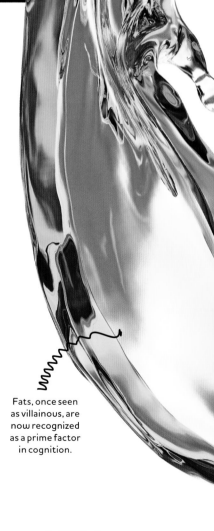

⁎ **THE RIGHT KINDS OF FAT ARE ESSENTIAL TO THE HEALTH OF YOUR BRAIN—FROM CELL MEMBRANES TO SYNAPSE FUNCTION—AND THAT HAS A DIRECT EFFECT ON LEARNING AND MEMORY.**

The human brain's relationship with fat is…complicated. Contradictions abound. For instance, the brain is a very fatty organ; studies have put the fat content of the brain at 60%. So you'd think the brain would gobble up fat as food to power its day-to-day functioning, right? Wrong. In fact, the abundant fat in the brain works not as fuel but as a kind of building block: Brain cells are wrapped in a sheath of fat called myelin, which protects and supports them and also provides insulation for electrical impulses traveling between cells. Most fats can't even get into the brain through the blood-brain barrier, which in terms of "fuel" lets through mainly glucose (the brain's favorite food) and ketones, an alternate fuel made by the liver that can serve as a backup when glucose is in short supply.

Many people might be surprised to learn that the brain can also make some of its own fat. Most of the saturated fats and monounsaturated fats in the brain are "homemade," according to Lisa Mosconi, PhD, author of *Brain Food: The Surprising Science of Eating for Cognitive Power*. But other fats need to come from outside sources, and they are so key to brain function that they're called "essential"

Fats, once seen as villainous, are now recognized as a prime factor in cognition.

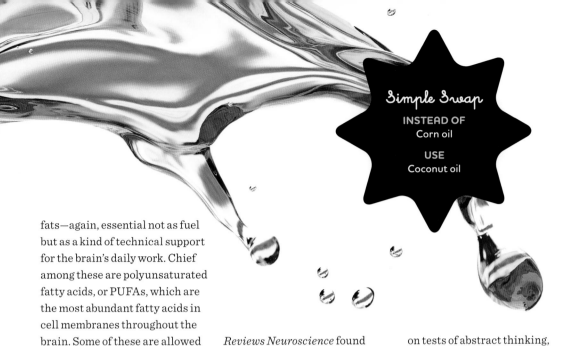

fats—again, essential not as fuel but as a kind of technical support for the brain's daily work. Chief among these are polyunsaturated fatty acids, or PUFAs, which are the most abundant fatty acids in cell membranes throughout the brain. Some of these are allowed to squeeze through the blood-brain barrier and circulate in the brain, and that's where the foods you eat play a very important role.

THE FATS YOUR BRAIN CRAVES

Omega-3 fatty acids—which cannot be manufactured by the brain, but must be consumed—have been shown in numerous studies to be the No. 1 nutrient to fight age-related cognitive decline and dementia. The most famous food source of omega-3s is, of course, fish and seafood, but these fatty acids are also found in some plant foods, such as flaxseeds and chia seeds. A study in the journal *Nature*

Reviews Neuroscience found that omega-3s are "crucial for maintaining [cell] membrane integrity" in the brain, along with the function of neurons and synapses. In real life, according to the study, that translates to low levels of omega-3 fatty acids being associated with an increased risk of "several mental disorders, including attention-deficit disorder, dyslexia, dementia, depression, bipolar and schizophrenia."

Another study, published in the journal *Neurology* in 2012, showed other stark real-world consequences to having low levels of omega-3 in the blood. Of the more than 1,500 study participants, those with blood levels in the lowest 25% had a lower total brain volume on MRIs, and also scored lower

on tests of abstract thinking, visual memory and focus.

On the other side, taking in plentiful omega-3s has been shown to benefit brain size and function. A study in the journal *Frontiers in Aging Neuroscience* found that older adults with higher blood levels of omega-3s had larger brain volume and greater "cognitive flexibility," i.e. mental functioning.

There is another form of PUFA, though, that may actually be overabundant in our food supply: omega-6 fatty acids. While these fats, found in foods such as vegetable oils and animal fats such as lard and chicken fat, are also essential, they work best in a specific balance with omega-3s—and can be dangerous at high levels. "Consuming a diet that is relatively higher in omega-6 compared to omega-3 contributes to systemic inflammation," says Laura LaChance, PhD, lecturer in brain and therapeutics at the University of Toronto. "That's because omega-6 fats lead to the production of pro-inflammatory cytokines, and omega-3s lead to the production of anti-inflammatory cytokines." If omega-6 gets a strong upper hand, inflammation (one of the brain's greatest enemies) can get out of control. Traditional diets like the Mediterranean diet, LaChance adds, "contain a ratio of approximately three-to-one omega-6 to omega-3. The modern American diet is closer to 20-to-one, which is a far cry from the diet we evolved to eat."

THE OILS YOU NEED

One reason those omega-6 fatty acids are so plentiful now in the American diet is that they abound in vegetable oils made

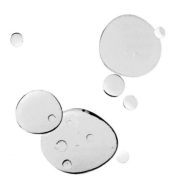

Rethink those so-called "healthy fats": Vegetable oils that are highly processed can throw off the balance of your omega-3 and -6 fatty acids.

from grapeseeds, canola, corn, peanuts and sunflower seeds—oils that have been promoted by public-health experts for years and are used heavily in restaurant and packaged-food preparation. Not only are Americans relying too much on these oils that have been touted as healthy, but many vegetable and seed oils, as currently formulated, go through intense processing at high heats (as opposed to oils that are cold-pressed, like olive and avocado), oxidizing them and making them toxic and inflammatory. Instead, stock your pantry with these cold-pressed oils, which are the backbone of traditional diets:

OLIVE OIL This mainly monounsaturated fat is antioxidant and anti-inflammatory, making it your brain's best friend. A study in the *Annals of Neurology* analyzed food surveys of more than 6,000 older women and found that the women with the most monounsaturated fat in their

diets performed the best on tests of memory and general cognition over time.

COCONUT OIL Although this oil is saturated, it's a type that operates differently in your body than animal-derived saturated fats. More than 50% of the fat in coconut oil is a type called medium-chain triglycerides (MCTs), which unlike longer-chain fats go straight to the liver and are more efficiently turned into energy. (For more on how MCTs work, see opposite page.)

WALNUT OIL Like the nuts that are used to source it, walnut oil is rich in brain-boosting omega-3 fatty acids, as well as other brain-friendly nutrients such as niacin, potassium and zinc.

AVOCADO OIL This delicious oil contains high levels of antioxidants, which fight free-radical damage in the brain, as well as monounsaturated fatty acids. A 2012 study found that these fatty acids helped protect nerve cells in the brain known as astrocytes, which support information-carrying nerves.

SESAME OIL This aromatic oil is high in omega-3 fatty acids, and also contains biologically active compounds called lignans, which have been shown to have neuroprotective effects and to reduce oxidative stress and the resulting damage in the brain.

IS MCT MAGIC?

THIS CONCENTRATED OIL HAS BEEN GETTING MAJOR BUZZ. HERE'S WHAT WE KNOW SO FAR ABOUT WHETHER THE HYPE LIVES UP TO THE REALITY.

Medium-chain triglycerides, or MCTs, act differently in the body than longer-chain fats, mainly because they break down more quickly. This means they can be more easily converted in the liver into ketones, an alternative energy source that can cross the blood-brain barrier. Several different oils contain some MCTs, including coconut and palm oils; MCT oil is made by extracting those MCTs into a nearly 100% concentration.

The ketone connection is what's causing the excitement, because there is preliminary evidence that ketones, a kind of "fat-replacement" compound, may benefit brain function. For instance, a small pilot study in the journal *BBA Clinical* in 2015 found that supplementing the diets of people with mild cognitive impairment with MCT oil increased blood levels of ketones and improved memory and performance on cognitive tests. According to the Alzheimer's Drug Discovery Foundation, people with cognitive decline or Alzheimer's disease have an impaired ability to use glucose, the brain's preferred fuel; ketones would supply an alternative energy source (and some say, perhaps a superior one). However, the group notes that study results have been mixed, and concludes "there exists no clinical data that MCTs promote long-term brain health."

That said, the risks of using MCT oil are low, and there has been no harm shown in adding some MCTs to your Bulletproof coffee as a possible boost to your brain. One important caveat: Your liver won't make ketones unless you're low on glucose stores, so to get the full benefit you should be on a low-carb or ketogenic diet. Since glucose is always the brain's "go-to" and favored energy source, it's unlikely that your brain will turn to using ketones unless it has run out of glucose. If you're seeking a ketone brain boost, cut the bread and starches.

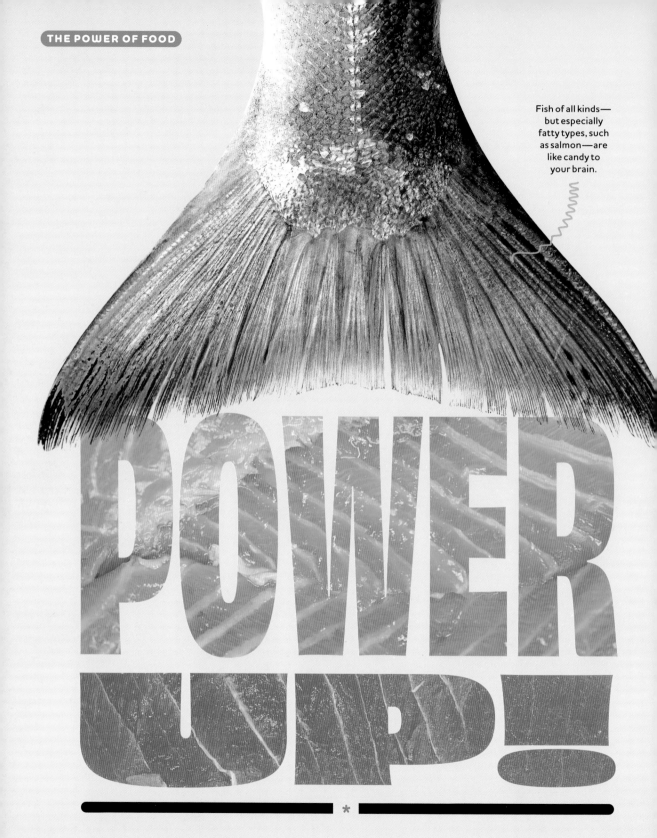

Fish of all kinds—but especially fatty types, such as salmon—are like candy to your brain.

POWER UP!

*

Of all the food groups that can supercharge the brain, protein may be the most intuitive. While we know that carbohydrates and fats play an important role in cognitive function, the image of protein is as a fount of neuron-driving energy. And although not all protein sources are necessarily brain-boosters (looking at you, salt-filled cured meats such as bacon and salami), it is indeed true that the building blocks of protein include some brain-friendly nutrients that aren't as readily available in other foods.

These include omega-3 fatty acids, the richest source of which is fatty fish; vitamin B12, only present in animal foods; other B vitamins such as thiamine and niacin; vitamins D and E; certain forms of iron; choline; and amino acids. Amino acids are organic compounds that combine to form proteins and are essential to brain function, according to Lisa Mosconi, PhD, associate director of the Alzheimer's Prevention Clinic at Weill Cornell Medical College New York-Presbyterian Hospital. As with fatty acids, some amino acids can be manufactured by the brain itself, while others, called "essential," must come from the diet. Amino acids are hard workers,

*

PROTEIN-PACKED FOODS ARE A KEY PART OF THE BRAIN-HEALTH PUZZLE. PUT THESE TOP SOURCES, FROM BOTH LAND AND SEA, ON THE MENU.

responsible for maintaining healthy tissues, assembling hormones, powering chemical reactions and even functioning as neurotransmitters—brain messengers that communicate and process information.

Protein is present in almost every food, though in larger or smaller amounts: more in animal products such as meat and eggs, somewhat less in plant-based sources such as legumes and nuts and small amounts in many fruits and vegetables. The most "complete" proteins, meaning they provide all 20-plus types of amino acids, needed to make new protein in the body, come from animal-based foods, while plant-based foods often lack one or more essential amino acids, according to the Harvard T.H. Chan School of Public Health. "Several essential nutrients for brain health, such as long chain omega-3s and B12, are only found in animal products," says Laura LaChance, PhD, lecturer in brain and therapeutics at the University of Toronto. "Animal products also contain absorbable iron and complete protein, in addition to many other essential nutrients such as choline."

That doesn't mean that you'll be protein (or amino acid) deficient if you're vegetarian or vegan, but it does mean you may need to take extra care (and, perhaps, a supplement or

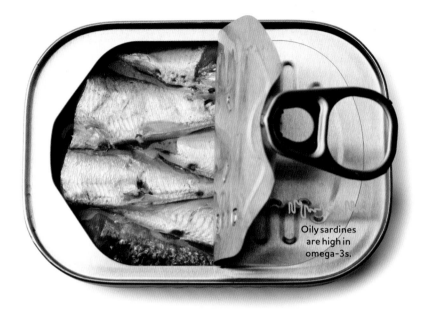

Oily sardines are high in omega-3s.

two—see the box on page 97 for more on vegan diets). Here's the lowdown on the specific brain benefits of the most common and popular protein foods.

FISH

Hands down, fish (especially wild-caught fatty fish such as salmon and tuna) wins the prize among protein-rich foods for boosting brain function. This is largely due to their high levels of omega-3 fatty acids, which have been strongly linked to cognitive health. To anthropologists, this isn't surprising: They hypothesize that fish, rather than the more difficult-to-acquire meat, was a key component of building brain size in early humans.

In a landmark article in the journal *Nature Reviews Neuroscience*, author Fernando Gómez-Pinilla, PhD, professor

and director of the Neurotrophic Research Laboratory at the University of California, Los Angeles, writes about the "abundant paleontological evidence" suggesting a direct relationship between access to food and brain size in humanoids, focusing specifically on a type of omega-3 fatty acid called docosahexaenoic acid (DHA). "It has been proposed that access to DHA during hominid evolution had a key role in increasing the brain/body-mass ratio," writes Gómez-Pinilla, who notes that DHA is the most abundant omega-3 in cell membranes in the brain. He describes a symbiotic relationship between nutrient and brain function: Archaeological evidence shows early man clustering around shorelines that supplied DHA-rich fish, which grew the human

brain over time because it supplied the precise nutrient our brains needed in order to develop and thrive.

Reams of animal and human studies have confirmed the importance of omega-3 fatty acids to brain function. For instance, a study in the *American Journal of Preventive Medicine* found that regular fish consumption is associated with a greater volume of gray matter in the brain; others show that higher fish consumption may affect brain structure and improve cognitive ability, delay the cognitive effects of aging and lower the risk of cardiovascular disease (which directly affects brain health).

EGGS

These bundles of nutrients have gone through their own public-relations crisis in recent decades, but the evidence is now placing them in the "yes" column. Packed with vitamins B6 and B12, both brain-boosting vitamins, they are also particularly rich in a nutrient called choline, which was recognized by the Institute

Some of the best brain food comes in a can— if you're talking sardines, tuna, salmon and other protein-rich fish.

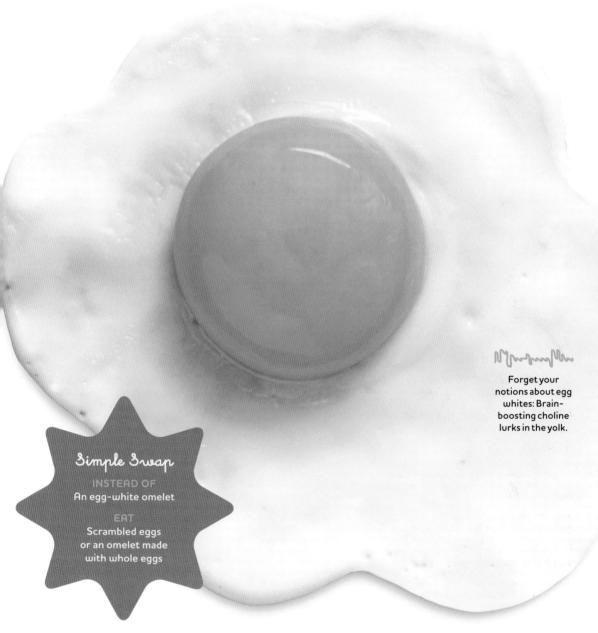

Forget your notions about egg whites: Brain-boosting choline lurks in the yolk.

of Medicine (now known as the National Academy of Medicine) as "essential" in 1998. Choline is used to produce fats that make up cell membranes, and is also converted into neurotransmitters like acetylcholine, which is crucial for memory and learning, according to Mosconi.

A study in the *British Journal of Nutrition* found that, in more than 2,000 participants in their 70s, those with higher choline levels had better cognitive functioning than those with low levels. But figures from the USDA show that most Americans aren't taking in the

recommended amount of this essential nutrient—and a chronic deficiency can contribute to neurological conditions like Alzheimer's disease. Choline is present in other sources, including beef liver, chicken and some plant sources like soy, but one of the easiest ways to take in enough is to simply include eggs in your diet (with the yolk, which is where the choline resides).

MEAT

Meats, including beef, lamb, pork and, to be expansive, poultry, have not always gotten the love that fish has for brain health. But in fact, eating the flesh of other animals brings along with it nutrients that are extremely important to brain health. And while some of these nutrients are available from other foods, certain key ones are not. Perhaps the most consequential of these is vitamin B12, a deficiency of which is associated with cognitive impairment in old age. Some studies have shown that the amount of B12 in a person's

Meat and fish are inextricably linked to human evolution, spurring greater brain size and better odds of survival.

blood later in life is correlated with their IQ, and that in the elderly, the brains of people with lower blood levels of B12 were six times more likely to be shrinking.

Another such nutrient is iron. The mineral is present in plant foods like spinach, but the form that is most readily absorbed by the body, called haem iron, is found only in animal proteins.

Research has linked iron levels to brain function, including a study finding that giving young women iron supplements led to significant intellectual gains. In those whose blood iron levels increased over the course of the study, performance on a cognitive test improved between five- and seven-fold. An amino acid called taurine is also plentiful in meat and seafood, and it is thought to be implicated in several brain processes, including regulating the number of neurons.

Bottom line, says LaChance: "Meat can be controversial these days, but unprocessed meats are a traditional food that we omnivores evolved to consume. That said, if you eat seafood, it's not a requirement to eat meat."

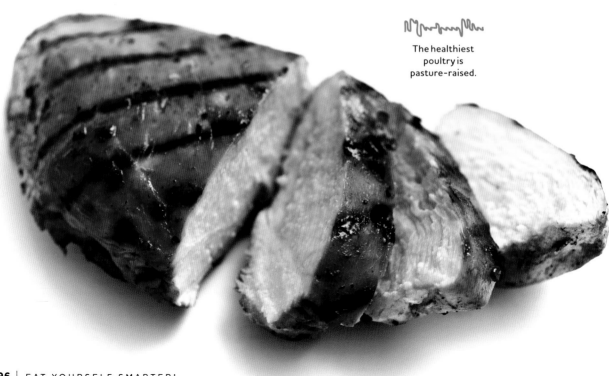

The healthiest poultry is pasture-raised.

Vegan Proteins

AVOIDING ANIMAL PRODUCTS?
YOU MAY NEED TO TAKE EXTRA
STEPS TO PROTECT YOUR BRAIN.

There's no way around it: Humans evolved as omnivores, and certain essential nutrients are found only, or largely, in animal foods. This has led some experts to be concerned about the nutritional status of vegans; Laura LaChance, PhD, even warns that "vegan diets require supplementation or can be lethal." Increasing numbers of people around the globe are vegan and appear to be thriving, but for optimal brain health, pay special attention to certain nutrients that may be lacking in a vegan diet.

Chief among these is vitamin B12, which has been closely linked to brain function. As people get older, they can have more difficulty absorbing vitamin B12 (which is only present in animal foods), just at the time that their brains are becoming more susceptible to dementia. Research has also linked a deficiency of B12 with cognitive decline. A study in England found that about half of vegans have low levels of B12. The most easily absorbable form of iron, another key brain nutrient, is also only present in animal products.

On the plus side, vegans tend to have healthier hearts, which is closely linked to brain health. One solution: supplements. Nutrients such as B12 and iron are easy to take in a multivitamin; other important nutrients, such as choline, creatine, carnosine and taurine, are bulkier and may require shopping for specific supplements. But

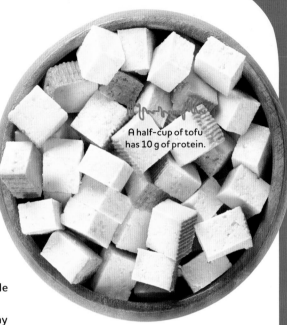

A half-cup of tofu
has 10 g of protein.

vegans can also strive to take in some of these nutrients in their plant form. Here's a list of foods, based on brain-boosting nutrients, to put on your healthy-vegan shopping list:

PROTEIN soy (including tofu and tempeh); nuts and seeds; legumes and beans; protein powders; certain grains (amaranth, barley, wheat berries)

CHOLINE brewer's yeast; shiitake mushrooms; wheat germ; quinoa; soy milk; certain beans (kidney, pinto); tofu; collard greens

OMEGA-3 FATTY ACIDS flaxseeds; chia seeds; Brussels sprouts; hempseeds; walnuts

IRON legumes (soybeans, lentils, chickpeas, black-eyed peas); nuts and seeds; potatoes; leafy greens (spinach, kale, Swiss chard, collard greens)

VITAMIN B6 chickpeas; potatoes; bananas; bulgur wheat; winter squash

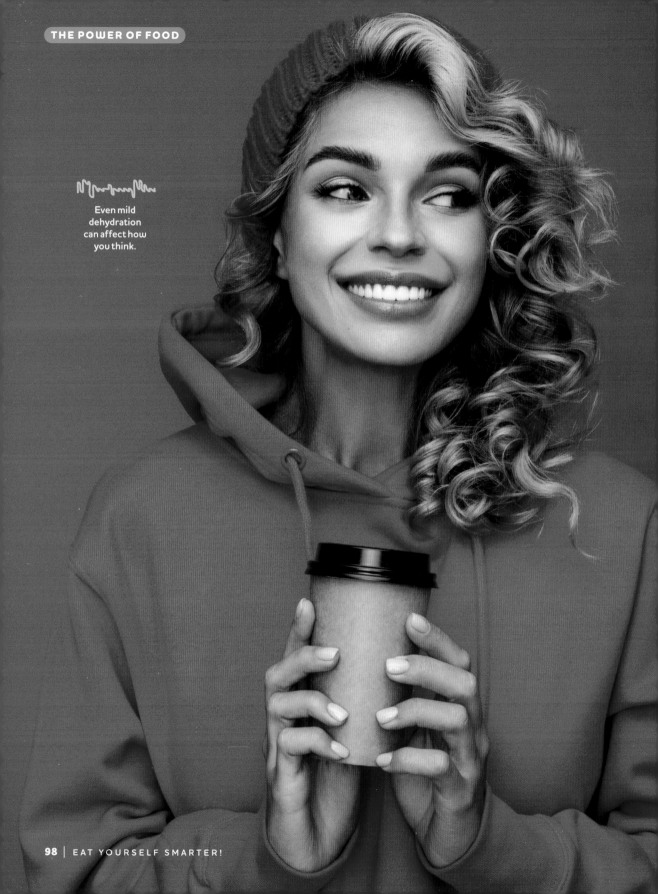

Even mild dehydration can affect how you think.

Drink to Your Brain

* NEURONS DO NOT LIVE BY FOOD ALONE. THE RIGHT FLUIDS, IN THE RIGHT AMOUNTS, KEEP YOUR NOGGIN'S CONNECTIONS FUNCTIONING, FLEXIBLE AND FINE-TUNED.

Quick: What's the best thing to drink for mental function? For many people, the self-evident answer might be one of those packaged beverages that tout words such as "energy" or "smart" on the label. But the real answer is so much simpler: water. Just plain old water. In part, that's because many of those commercial drinks are packed with sugar, which is one of your brain's sworn enemies, due to its inflammatory properties. But it's also because pure water performs a myriad of absolutely essential tasks in the brain, from carrying oxygen to being involved in every chemical reaction that occurs.

Water is as central to the life of a brain as it is to the life of a planet (which is why, when it comes to seeking extraterrestrial life, we scour the solar system looking for evidence of water). Your brain, by weight, is about 80% water, compared to 60% in the rest of your body. While humans can survive weeks without food, we can go at most a few days without water. The slightest dehydration, even just a 3% to 4% decrease in water intake, can lead quickly to fatigue, mental confusion and disorientation. And yet, studies have found that a majority of Americans are chronically dehydrated without realizing it.

That daily, low-level or barely noticeable dehydration takes a toll on your mental health and functioning. A study in *The Journal of Nutrition* found that being dehydrated by less than 2% lowered participants' mood and ability to concentrate; another study, in the *British Journal of Nutrition*, found that mild dehydration "induced adverse changes in vigilance and working memory, and increased tension/anxiety and fatigue."

Dehydration can even affect the brain's volume of gray matter and white matter, according to a study in the journal *PLOS One*, making the brain look—at least temporarily—similar to the brains of people with mild cognitive impairment or Alzheimer's. While the effects of dehydration can be reversed by increasing water intake, these results are especially alarming because aging alters sensitivity to thirst, making older adults more vulnerable to being in a constant state of dehydration.

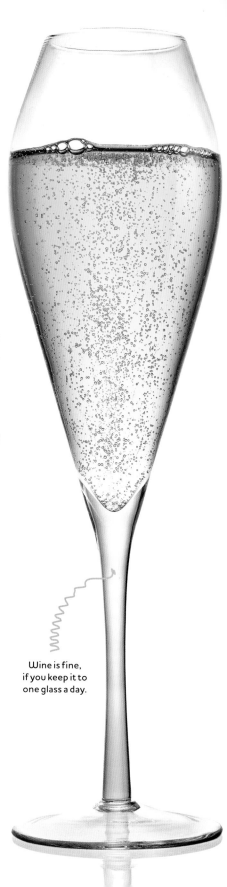

Wine is fine, if you keep it to one glass a day.

On the plus side, drinking enough water can quickly improve your mental function. A 2013 study in the journal *Frontiers in Human Neuroscience* had participants take a battery of cognitive tests on two different occasions: once after a night of fasting when no water was given, and again after a night of fasting when about 16 ounces of water were offered during the test. They showed significantly better results and faster response times after drinking the water. So, simple rule No. 1: Step up your water game. Shoot for eight 8-ounce glasses a day, and adjust that according to your personal needs. If you're physically active or you live in a warm climate, for example, you may well need more than that. And remember that if you feel thirsty, that means you're already somewhat dehydrated.

Water is a baseline step, though. You'll encounter many other drinks during the course of your day, some that will add brain benefits and others that can throw your brain off course. Read on for the winners and losers.

COFFEE AND TEA

Coffee is one of those scientific oddities: Researchers keep trying to find bad things to say about it and coming up short. From lowering cancer risk to boosting mood, benefits have continually cropped up in research over the past couple of decades.

First, two superlatives: Coffee has been described as the world's No. 1 source of antioxidants (it is made, after all, from the fruit of the coffee plant; a 2013 study in the journal *Antioxidants* identified numerous polyphenols in green coffee beans, some of which are actually amplified by the roasting process); and its most active ingredient, caffeine, has been called the most popular psychoactive substance across the globe.

In the short term, almost everyone knows from experience

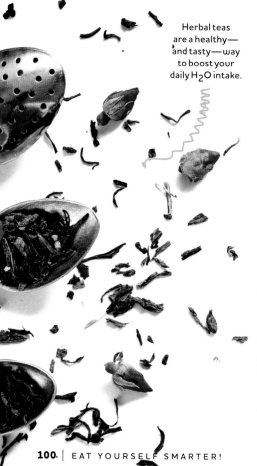

Herbal teas are a healthy— and tasty—way to boost your daily H_2O intake.

A study found that whether people drank several smaller cups of coffee over a few hours or one big cup, the caffeine led to better mental performance.

that coffee and other caffeine-containing beverages, like tea, give a fast-acting energy boost. In part, this is because caffeine blocks an inhibitory neurotransmitter in the brain called adenosine, which allows other neurotransmitters such as norepinephrine and dopamine to increase, upping the firing of neurons. Many studies have documented caffeine's ability to improve memory, task vigilance, energy levels, reaction time and general cognitive function.

If you are a regular caffeine consumer, these short-term boosts play out in significant longer-term health benefits, many of which are closely tied to brain health. For instance, studies have shown that coffee drinkers have a significantly lower risk of developing type 2 diabetes, a disease that on its own makes you twice as likely to get Alzheimer's down the road. And numerous other studies, including one in the *European*

Journal of Neurology, have found that caffeine intake is associated with a significantly lower risk of developing Alzheimer's disease. Coffee drinkers also have a risk reduction ranging from 32% to 60% of getting Parkinson's disease—the second-most common neurodegenerative condition after Alzheimer's—perhaps because of its effect on dopamine-generating neurons.

Then there is coffee's effect on mood and depression. A study of long-term coffee drinkers in the *Archives of Internal Medicine* found that they were 53% less likely to die by suicide than non-coffee drinkers, and a Harvard study in 2011 showed that women who drank coffee had

a 20% lower risk overall of becoming depressed.

Tea shares many of coffee's antioxidant and caffeine-related benefits, and adds in some of its own—especially green tea. It is rich in L-theanine, an amino acid that can cross the blood-brain barrier and influence the activity of neurotransmitters. It's also packed with polyphenols, which fight oxidative stress and damage in the brain. Green tea has been shown to improve working memory and attention and lower the risk of cognitive impairment. Epidemiologists have looked at cultures where green tea is most popular and found much lower

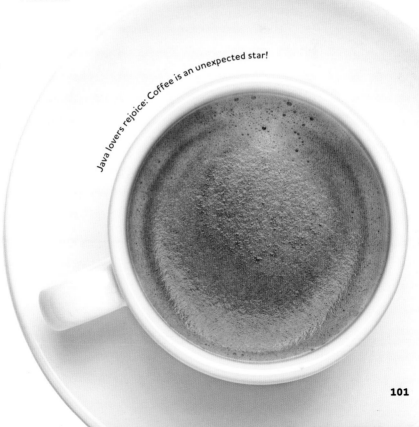

Java lovers rejoice: Coffee is an unexpected star!

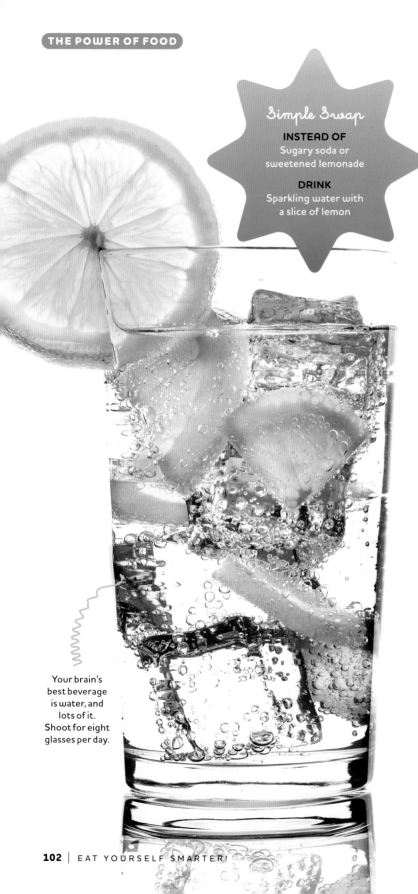

Simple Swap

INSTEAD OF
Sugary soda or
sweetened lemonade

DRINK
Sparkling water with
a slice of lemon

Your brain's
best beverage
is water, and
lots of it.
Shoot for eight
glasses per day.

rates of dementia than in parts
of the world where green tea-
drinking is less common.

ALCOHOL

The effects of alcohol on the brain
are a distinctly mixed bag—about
as varied as the different forms
of booze, from whiskey to wine.
Red wine (again, like coffee,
made from polyphenol-rich
fruit) is very high in "antioxidant
activity," according to a study in
the journal *Antioxidants*, coming
in between coffee and green tea in
a ranking, and has been linked to
cardiovascular health. But unlike
those caffeine-filled drinks, the
benefits of red wine have a fairly
low ceiling: Go beyond one or two
glasses and the risks outweigh
the benefits. Numerous studies
show that the antioxidant- and
anti-inflammatory-related
health boosts from a glass or
two are quickly eradicated by
overindulgence.

A study in *The BMJ* found a
"dose dependent" relationship
between alcohol consumption
and damage to the brain,
including atrophy in the
hippocampus (the center
of learning and memory)
and an accelerated rate of
cognitive decline. That matches
widespread research showing
that prolonged alcohol use can
have long-term effects on brain
function. Just consider the
phenomenon of an alcoholic
"blackout," in which the brain
is temporarily unable to store

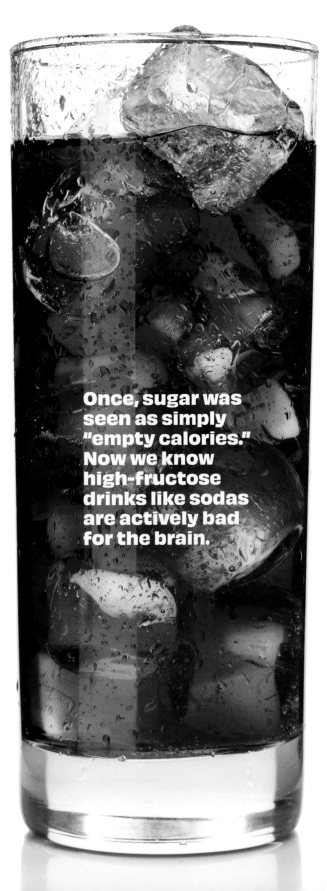

Once, sugar was seen as simply "empty calories." Now we know high-fructose drinks like sodas are actively bad for the brain.

memories after having several drinks on one occasion. That's a direct illustration of how the toxins that lead to "intoxication" block function in the parts of the brain that govern memory. Heavy drinkers also often have a deficiency of thiamine (vitamin B1), an essential nutrient that facilitates the brain's uptake of glucose, its primary fuel. Abnormalities in glucose uptake and metabolism are a common feature of Alzheimer's disease.

Bottom line: If you do want to drink alcohol, choose a glass of red wine over spirits, and keep it to one a day, tops.

SUGARY DRINKS

This category includes healthy-sounding beverages like sports and energy drinks—and even 100% fruit juices (which, unlike a piece of whole fruit, deliver a big dose of sugar with no fiber to slow its effect on blood sugar). Not surprisingly, sweetened sodas, which are packed with high-fructose corn syrup, are the worst offenders. Sugar is increasingly seen as the culprit in systemic inflammation, which raises cardiovascular risk and is strongly implicated in cognitive decline. For superior brain health, plan on deleting this entire category from your lifestyle. (For more on how this relationship works, and why these drinks should be off the menu completely, see page 104.)

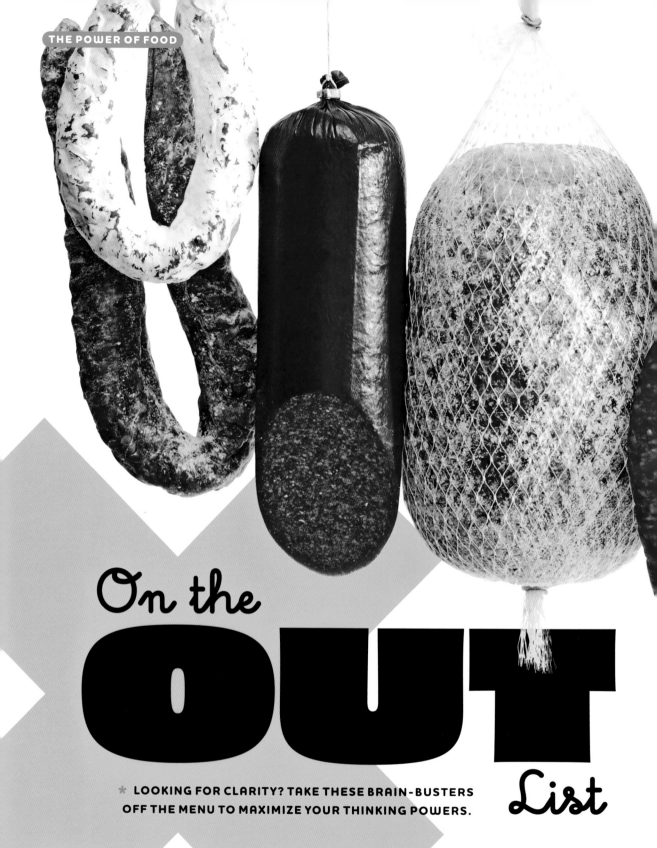

On the OUT List

* LOOKING FOR CLARITY? TAKE THESE BRAIN-BUSTERS OFF THE MENU TO MAXIMIZE YOUR THINKING POWERS.

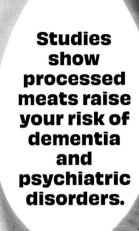

Studies show processed meats raise your risk of dementia and psychiatric disorders.

Almost everything in this book is about what to eat to make your brain work better, feel happier and last longer, well into old age. But there is one other extremely important part of the puzzle: the foods that actively work *against* those goals. Admittedly, many of these are popular items that have masqueraded as "feel-good foods" or comfort foods—among them chips, microwavable snacks, doughnuts and hot dogs. But once you know more about how certain foods act in your body and brain, the less comforting you may find them. And their very popularity, say

Swap out sausage for a piece of plain pork with tasty seasonings.

experts, is part of the problem. "The standard American diet, which people abbreviate as SAD, is high in refined carbohydrates and sugar," says Laura LaChance, PhD, a researcher and lecturer in brain and therapeutics at the University of Toronto. "The SAD also tends to be nutrient-poor—which has led to high rates of nutrient deficiencies

in North America—and low in antioxidants." The damage from those tendencies, LaChance says, includes blood sugar dysregulation that contributes to insulin resistance and inflammation, as well as greater oxidative stress, aka free radicals. Both inflammation and oxidative stress are harmful to brain function over time.

In many ways, a brain-*un*healthy diet is the evil twin—or fun house-mirror version—of a brain-healthy diet. It contains trans and saturated fats in place of monounsaturated fats and omega-3 fatty acids; highly refined carbs in place of minimally processed whole grains like brown rice; sweetened beverages in place of water and tea; and artificial flavors in place of vitamin-rich natural phytochemicals. The good news is that the fix is clear: By putting the following foods on your personal "out" list, you can take a giant step toward better cognitive function.

PROCESSED FOODS

First, a simple definition: "Processed" foods means anything that comes in a box, bag, can or freezer pack. There are a few exceptions, of course; plain frozen vegetables or fruits with no added ingredients are fine (and can make a great smoothie), as are a flash-frozen fillet of wild salmon or a box of brown rice. But if you think in terms of whole foods that you cook yourself—a baked potato rather than packaged french fries or chips; fresh spinach sauteed in olive oil in place of a frozen or take-out creamed spinach side dish—you're already on the road to a sharper brain.

That's not just because fresh foods retain more of the vital nutrients that feed your neurons, but also, and even more importantly, because of the other, unwelcome ingredients added to processed foods to keep them shelf-stable for unnatural amounts of time. High on that list are unhealthy fats (such as saturated fats and trans fatty

acids) and large amounts of salt and sugar to pump up flavor (because the older a food is, the less flavor it has). Processed foods that are high in fat and sugar have been shown to have an almost immediate effect on brain function—and not in a good way.

A study in the *Journal of Cerebral Blood Flow & Metabolism* compared rats on a normal rat-chow diet to rats eating food supplemented with lard (saturated fat) and sugar. In just seven days, the fat-and-sugar rats showed changes to the hippocampus, the region of the brain devoted to memory and learning. There, the neurons' dendrites—the long, branch-like structures that transmit electrical signals in the brain—were shorter and thinner, and they also had fewer synapses, the tiny structures at the end

of dendrites that help neurons communicate. At the same time, glial cells in the hippocampus had grown larger and become activated, a sign of increased inflammation. So in just one week, the hippocampus wasn't communicating as well as it should, and was also becoming inflamed, further impairing communication. To add insult to injury, the fat-and-sugar rats also became obese and insulin-resistant.

Other studies have turned up similar results: Researchers have fed rats a "junk food" diet high in saturated fat and sugar and found a "decline in cognitive performance and reduced hippocampal levels of synaptic plasticity." The rats performed worse on learning tasks, because their diet was doing damage to their neurons.

Inflammation caused by sugar can damage both heart and brain.

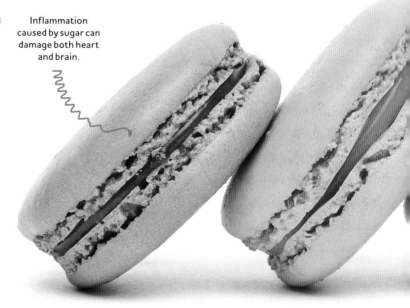

FAST FOODS

OK, so eating out of boxes, cans and microwave pouches is out, but a fresh-cooked fast-food burger can't be *that* bad, right? Wrong. It may be no surprise that fast food isn't health food, but beyond its propensity for expanding your waistline, drive-through specialties have been shown to have a specific effect on the brain and learning. First, fast food is nutrient-poor, denuded of brain favorites such as omega-3 fatty acids, vitamins B, C and E, and the many antioxidant and anti-inflammatory ingredients that are plentiful in, say, the Mediterranean diet.

Even worse, though, is what it does have: typically lots of sugar and salt (read on) and a big dose of unhealthy fats. Most fast food is fried in either saturated fat or vegetable oils—which have

Think you can make healthy fast-food choices? Even a taco salad at Taco Bell contains almost an entire day's limit for saturated fat intake.

been sold to consumers for years under the guise of "healthy fats," but which actually become oxidized under high heat conditions. That oxidation lets loose free radicals (unstable particles that can damage neurons) in the brain. Various studies have linked high intake of fast food to lower scores on cognitive and memory tests.

SUGAR

Along with being a major component in other "out list" foods like convenience and fast foods, this nutrient is in a category of one for its destructiveness to the brain. That's in part because sugar is highly inflammatory, and inflammation in the brain disrupts neuronal and synaptic function—and has even been linked to Alzheimer's disease.

A high-sugar diet also messes with your insulin function and what researchers call "brain energy metabolism," meaning the ability of your brain to get the best fuel. A study in *The Journal of Physiology* found that disruptions in insulin receptors due to a high-sugar diet affected synaptic plasticity—the ability of your synapses to communicate and "learn" from experience. The result: "impaired cognitive function." Insulin also increases blood flow, and other studies show that insulin resistance (an effect of a high-sugar diet) can reduce blood flow in the brain and impair memory function.

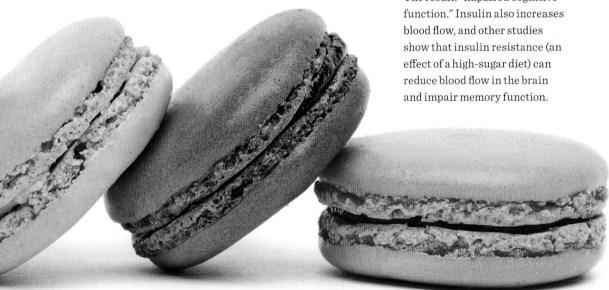

SALT

Another ubiquitous ingredient in processed and fast foods, salt, is also emerging as a direct enemy of the brain. It had been thought that salt might be bad for your brain because it's implicated in high blood pressure—and anything that constricts delivery and circulation of blood in the brain is bad news. But a study in the journal *Nature Neuroscience* in 2018 shows that salt inflicts damage to the brain in a much more primary way.

Researchers found that mice which had been on a high-salt diet for eight weeks showed marked reductions in cerebral blood flow in two areas of the brain involved in learning and memory, the

U.S. guidelines suggest no more than about one teaspoon of salt per day, but most Americans far exceed that level of intake.

cortex and the hippocampus— even though they didn't develop high blood pressure. The good news: Mice that were then returned to a regular diet for four weeks had their cerebral blood flow return to normal. But the ones who stayed on the high-salt diet developed dementia, performing significantly worse on tests and even in daily living activities like nest-building.

Salt has been shown to use another pathway to cognitive impairment, as well. In a 2019 study in *Nature*, it was found that a high-salt diet affected the stability of tau proteins in neurons. Not only does tau provide structure for the physical scaffolding, or cytoskeleton, of neurons to support their function, but one of the hallmarks of Alzheimer's disease is when it goes haywire. People with that most common form of dementia have a buildup of two proteins, tau and another protein called B-amyloid, in their brains, which disrupts communication between neurons.

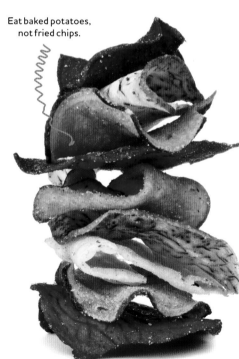

Eat baked potatoes, not fried chips.

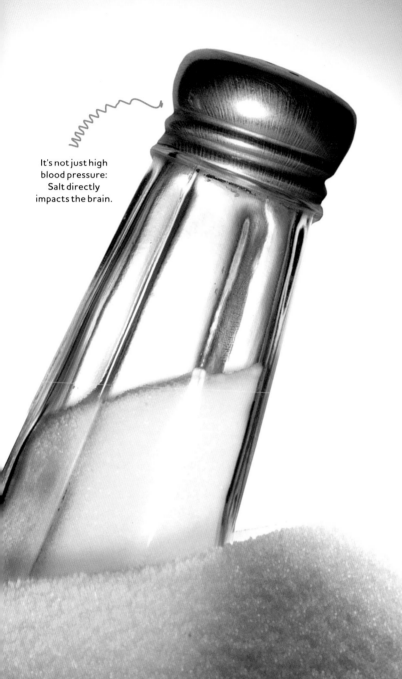

It's not just high blood pressure: Salt directly impacts the brain.

Brain Enemies

THESE FOODS ARE INFLAMMATORY AND HAVE BEEN SHOWN TO HAVE DELETERIOUS EFFECTS ON BRAIN FUNCTION, SO LIMIT YOUR INTAKE.

FRIED FOODS french fries, doughnuts, fried chicken, mozzarella sticks, egg rolls

JUNK FOODS fast foods, convenience meals, chips, pretzels

PROCESSED MEATS bacon, beef jerky, salami, hot dogs, smoked meats

REFINED CARBS white bread, pasta, crackers, tortillas, cookies, cakes, pies

SUGAR-SWEETENED BEVERAGES soda, sports and energy drinks

TRANS FATS shortening, partially hydrogenated vegetable oil, margarine—avoid these entirely

Can PILLS Do the Job?

* SUPPLEMENT MAKERS WANT YOU TO THINK SO — BUT EVIDENCE IS HARD TO FIND. HERE'S WHAT THE SCIENCE IS SHOWING.

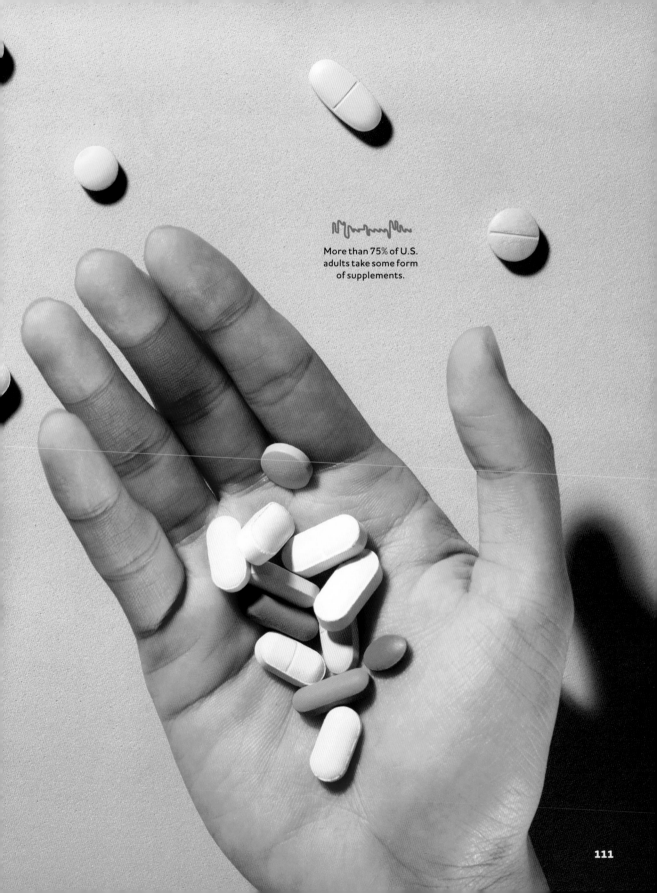

More than 75% of U.S.
adults take some form
of supplements.

True to the enduring American hope of finding a shortcut to health, a substantial number of adults around the country have looked beyond food to pills as a boost to their brains.

After all, the thinking goes, if omega-3-rich fish is so good for that all-important organ, why not just cut to the chase and swallow a capsule of concentrated omega-3s? And what about adding in those pills made from mysterious or "newly discovered" nutrients that claim to miraculously improve your memory?

Nearly one in four people over age 18 in the U.S. takes a supplement to maintain or improve brain health, or to delay or reverse dementia, according to the 2019 AARP Brain Health and Dietary Supplements Survey. And demand for memory supplements is growing: Sales in the U.S. nearly doubled from 2006 to 2015, when the market for such brain-boosters reached $643 million. The question of whether they are worth the money, though, is still largely unanswered.

"People take 'brain-boosting supplements' in hopes of reducing the decline in cognitive function as they age," says Paul M. Coates, PhD, vice president of the American Society for Nutrition and former director of the Office of Dietary Supplements at the National Institutes of Health (NIH). "But the evidence is weak to nonexistent that any of them work." Read on for a closer look at the pros and cons.

BEHIND THE LABEL

"Dietary supplement" is an umbrella term that includes everything from vitamins, minerals and amino acids to botanicals (including herbs) and enzymes. They're sold as pills, capsules, tablets, powders, liquids, even food bars. For the most part, though, "supplement" refers to vitamins, minerals and multivitamins. Many common supplements make claims for brain-boosting benefits, based on varying amounts of research

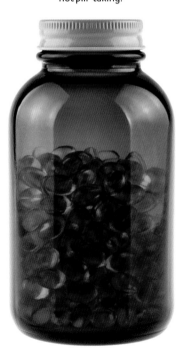

Most omega-3 studies look at fish-eating, not pill-taking.

suggesting that eating a diet rich in these nutrients may be good for the brain. These include nutrients such as omega-3 fatty acids; ginseng, ginkgo biloba, and resveratrol; vitamins A, B, D, E; and trace minerals such as zinc.

For its survey, AARP collaborated with the Global Council on Brain Health (GCBH), an independent group of scientists, doctors, scholars and policy experts from around the world. After reviewing the brain-health supplements' potential effectiveness, the GCBH wasn't able to endorse any ingredient, product or supplement designed for brain health. The best way to get your nutrients for brain health? From a wholesome diet, the GCBH concluded. The science on whether getting these nutrients through a dietary supplement yields the same benefits as food is, at best, soft to medium-hard.

Meanwhile, a new arena has opened in the brain-supplement market, centered on less-familiar ingredients, and some of these have watchdogs concerned. A case in point: the widely advertised Prevagen. An estimated 1 million people in the U.S. have taken Prevagen, which promises to improve your memory, clear your head and sharpen your mind. Never mind that the main ingredient is the synthetic version of a protein found in jellyfish (apoaequorin). Or that the only

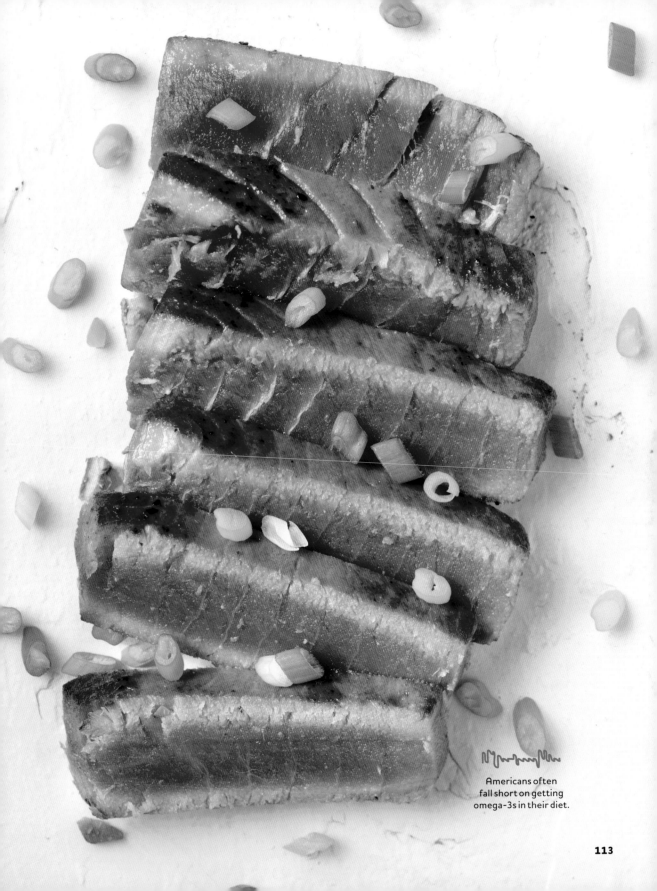

Americans often
fall short on getting
omega-3s in their diet.

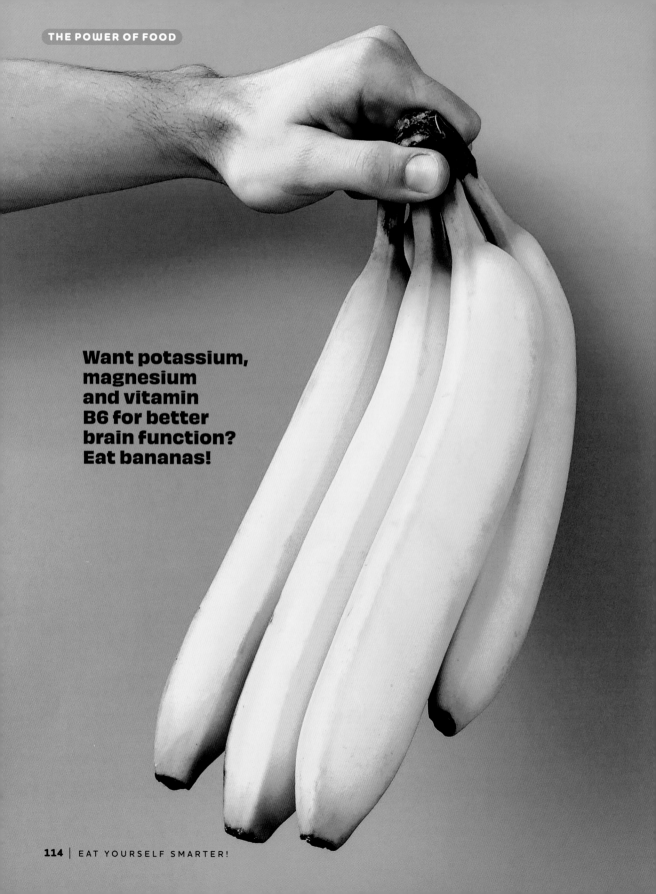

Want potassium, magnesium and vitamin B6 for better brain function? Eat bananas!

"proof" that it works is a study sponsored by Quincy Bioscience Manufacturing—the company that makes the supplement.

That study, published in a 2016 issue of *Advances in Mind-Body Medicine*, looked at the effect of Prevagen on cognitive function in adults ages 40 and older who had concerns about their brain health. The findings suggest only minimal improvement in memory, despite the company's claims to the contrary.

The U.S. Food and Drug Administration (FDA) and Federal Trade Commission (FTC) finally stepped in and said, essentially, enough already with the fraudulent claims. Enough, too, of keeping consumers in the dark about the potential risks—including seizures and strokes—of taking Prevagen. Ultimately, seven lawsuits were filed by consumers over allegations of false advertising. In early 2020, Quincy agreed to compensate consumers who'd bought Prevagen with payments of up to $70.

Prevagen is hardly the only dubious dietary supplement promising to ward off cognitive decline. In 2019, the FDA and FTC sent warning letters to a number of companies for making what they said were false or unsubstantiated health claims. Specifically: Gold Crown Natural Products was peddling its colostrum and melatonin supplements as a cure for Alzheimer's; TEK Naturals said

Ginseng root is a traditional remedy in China.

its Mind Ignite supplement was "clinically shown to help diseases of the brain such as Alzheimer's and even dementia"; and Pure Nootropics was—and still is—selling a number of supplements, all of which have authentic-sounding ingredients, like uridine monophosphate, which claims to support overall brain function; lion's mane mushrooms, which purport to boost memory, mood and focus; and pyrroloquinoline quinone, said to promote cognitive function while aging.

THE PSYCHOLOGY OF SUPPLEMENTS

So why do so many people take supplements if the health benefits are negligible—or nonexistent—for the average healthy person? "In national surveys, people report that they take dietary supplements for a variety of reasons, but generally and mainly to improve health, maintain health, supplement their diet and prevent health problems," says Paul R. Thomas, EdD, RDN, a scientific consultant to the NIH Office of Dietary Supplements. "Supplements of vitamins and minerals can help ensure that people get recommended intakes of these

nutrients, especially if they do not eat as well as they know they should." But many people take supplements to go beyond that baseline, hoping the pills will actively improve their health—including their brain function—over time, and as they age.

That hope may be due to the rise of what a 2019 report in *JAMA* dubbed pseudomedicine: the practice of using supplements and medical interventions that are legal and often promoted as scientifically supported treatments for dementia and brain health, even though they haven't been proven effective. As the article points out, these supplements come off sounding legit because they quote research to back up their claims—even though the studies cited are often done in animals (meaning the results are considered by scientists to be preliminary, at best) and many of those done in humans

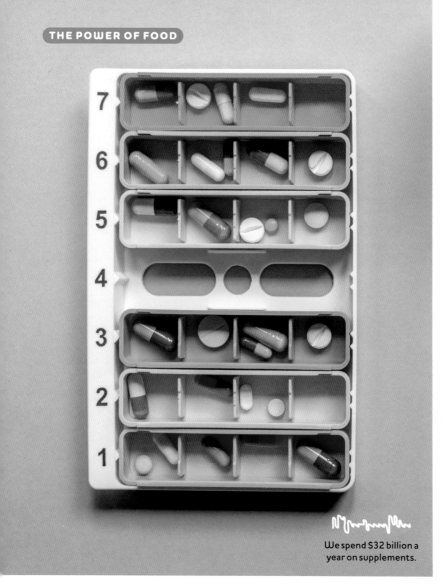

We spend $32 billion a year on supplements.

dietary supplements that are adulterated, either intentionally or unintentionally, with prescription medications or unapproved drugs," says Thomas. "By definition, they are not dietary supplements—laws prohibit such adulteration—but products masquerading as dietary supplements."

In fact, a 2020 study in *Neurology Clinical Practice* found that over-the-counter cognitive enhancement supplements may contain a number of unapproved drugs. Researchers "uncovered numerous examples of products containing dangerous or illegal ingredients; others have, too," says Coates. "Consumers deserve to know that the products they purchase are safe under normal conditions of use. For the great majority of products in the marketplace, that is true. Sadly, there are a few instances where it is not."

In any case, your best bet is to check with your doctor before adding any supplements, brain-supporting or otherwise, to your daily regimen, says Thomas. "This is especially important if you are taking any prescription medicines, because some ingredients in dietary supplements can negatively interact with them. When you take a new product, pay attention to what effects it may be having on you—those you hope for, and others that may be unintended and possibly harmful."

haven't been published in a peer-reviewed scientific journal.

Even so, the average consumer might assume that over-the-counter supplements wouldn't be on the market if they weren't safe and effective. In a 2019 survey by Pew Charitable Trusts, more than half the respondents were under the impression that the FDA either tests supplements for safety or approves them before they're made available to consumers. Neither is true. Instead, the FDA relies on reporting by the companies and consumers, as well as its own inspections, to spot potential problems once supplements are on the market. (The agency has since announced plans to change the way it regulates dietary supplements by beefing up its level of oversight.)

"There are products on the market labeled as

WORTH A TRY?

IF YOU STILL WANT TO GIVE PILLS THE BENEFIT OF THE DOUBT, USE THIS RESOURCE.

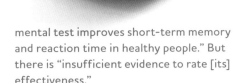

Be cautious before trying ginkgo.

A good way to get up to speed on the science-backed benefits of a given supplement is to check the National Institutes of Health's Office of Dietary Supplements' fact sheets (ods.od.nih.gov). They provide a snapshot of what government scientists have concluded, so far, about safety and efficacy. Some excerpts about popular brain supplements:

ACETYL-L-CARNITINE "Research in aged rats found supplementation with high doses of acetyl-L-carnitine and alpha-lipoic acid (an antioxidant) to reduce mitochondrial decay. The animals also moved about more and improved their performance on memory-requiring tasks. At present there are no equivalent studies…in humans. However, a meta-analysis of double-blind, placebo-controlled studies suggests that supplements of acetyl-L-carnitine may improve mental function and reduce deterioration in older adults with mild cognitive impairment and Alzheimer's disease."

GINKGO "Consumers should be aware that studies have not consistently demonstrated that ginkgo improves brain function. National Toxicology Program findings showing that both rats and mice develop cancer after long-term use should also be taken into consideration. Additionally, ginkgo has been shown to interact with other drugs, which can increase or decrease their effects."

GINSENG "Early research shows that taking American ginseng one to six hours before a mental test improves short-term memory and reaction time in healthy people." But there is "insufficient evidence to rate [its] effectiveness."

OMEGA-3 FATTY ACIDS "Some research indicates that people who eat more seafood may have a reduced risk of cognitive decline. However, omega-3 supplements haven't been shown to help prevent cognitive impairment or Alzheimer's disease or to improve symptoms of these conditions. For example, a large NIH-sponsored study completed in 2015 indicated that taking EPA and DHA supplements did not slow cognitive decline in older adults."

VITAMIN E "Several studies have investigated whether vitamin E supplements might help older adults remain mentally alert and active as well as prevent or slow the decline of mental function and Alzheimer's disease. So far, the research provides little evidence that taking vitamin E supplements can help healthy people, or people with mild mental functioning problems."

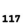

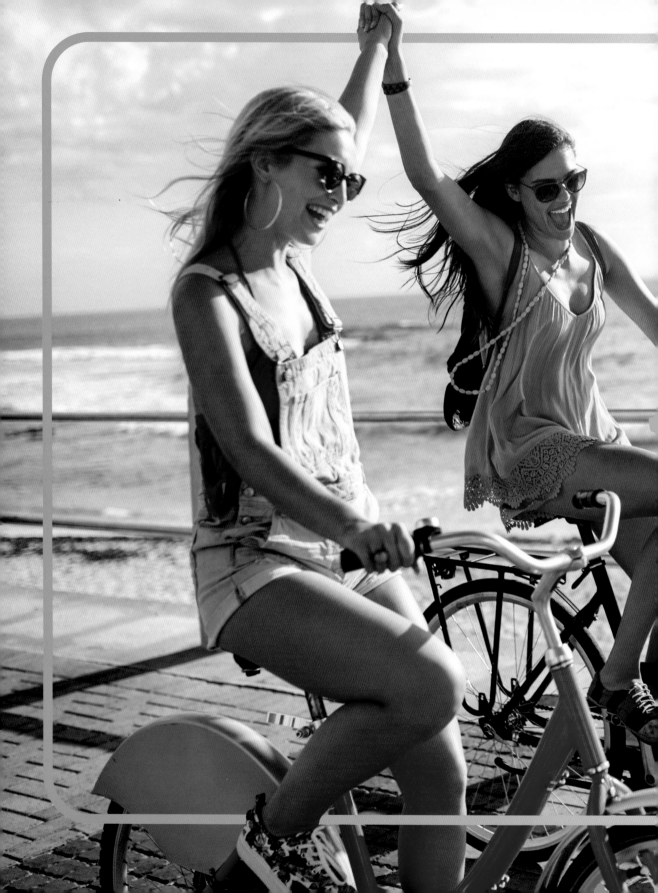

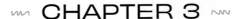

CHAPTER 3
Easy
BRAIN
Boosters

FROM HANGING WITH FRIENDS TO GETTING A
GOOD NIGHT'S SLEEP AND REGULAR EXERCISE,
THERE ARE PLENTY OF WAYS TO STAY SHARP.

Why We Need FRIENDS

✳ HOW SOCIAL CONNECTIONS MAKE US SMARTER AND STRENGTHEN THE BRAIN.

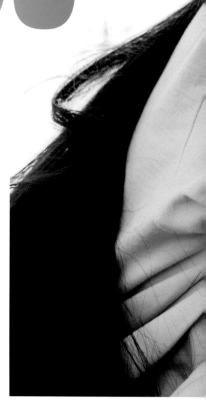

We imagine that love for our family and friends feeds our souls and not our brains. But human connection fuels brain development, protects brain health and is the likely reason our brains are so big and capable to begin with.

Studies of orphans have shown how detrimental a lack of a healthy attachment and physical closeness to caregivers are to a baby's cognitive and emotional development. Recently, a study published in *Science* reported that social interaction in early life has irreversible effects on the growth of connections in the brain's prefrontal cortex. Missing that window of opportunity has lifelong repercussions.

Psychologist Michael Tomasello has done groundbreaking studies with both chimps and toddlers supporting his theory that the ability to cooperate—a likely precursor to friendship formation—is what sets humans apart from the apes. British anthropologist Robin Dunbar proposed the "social brain

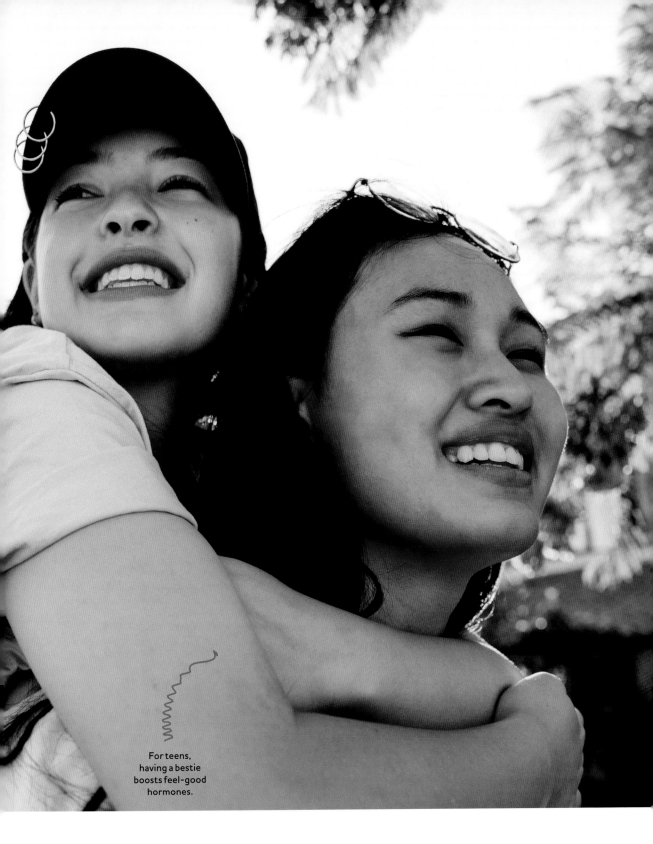

For teens, having a bestie boosts feel-good hormones.

hypothesis," which posits that human intelligence evolved not primarily to solve problems out in the world but rather to navigate the complex social world of friends and relatives.

Dunbar discovered that the size of a primate's brain is correlated with the size of the social group within which its species typically lives. The magic number for humans—extrapolated from our average brain size—is 150. "In effect we have five intimate friends (or relatives), 15 close friends, 50 good friends and 150 friends," Dunbar says. One hundred and 50 also corresponds with the average size of tribes we lived in when our brains were evolving. (Funnily enough, the number of Twitter users people tend to interact with before becoming overwhelmed is 150.)

In one study, Dunbar found that the volume of a subject's orbital prefrontal cortex correlates with the size of his social circle as well as his ability to comprehend others' state of mind while interacting with them, a skill called "mentalizing ability." Another research team found a correlation between the size of the amygdala, a brain region that processes emotional stimuli, and both the size and the complexity of a person's social network.

A neuroimaging study found feelings of exclusion can affect an area of the brain that's also responsible for the sensation of physical pain.

A BRAIN MADE FOR FRIENDS

Our brains are now forced to adapt to a very new social order, however. "In traditional societies, everyone's 150 overlaps with everyone else's, so everyone knows everyone else," Dunbar says. "That gives the community a great degree of structural strength. What has happened with modern, post-World War II economic mobility has been that our social networks have become fragmented and geographically dispersed. This gives us more freedom, certainly. The cost we pay is that networks are less mutually supporting."

Matthew Lieberman, a neuroscientist at UCLA and the author of *Social: Why Our Brains Are Wired to Connect*, has discovered that whenever we're not actively trying to do something, our brain organizes

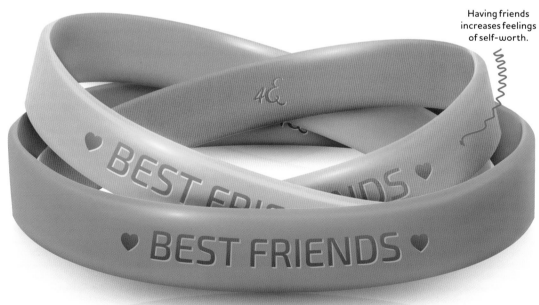

Having friends increases feelings of self-worth.

BEST FRIENDS

♥ BEST FRIENDS ♥

Keep Your Friends, Keep Your Health

MORE THAN JUST GOOD FUN, HAVING A NETWORK YOU CAN RELATE TO CAN HAVE A VERY REAL POSITIVE EFFECT ON YOUR BODY AND MIND.

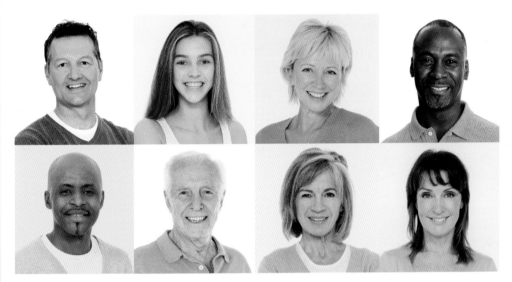

Evidence that positive relationships translate to better health is so strong that encouraging friendships should be a health-care initiative. Consider the weight-friendship connection: In a network analysis, researchers Nicholas Christakis and James Fowler found that if a person's friend becomes obese, it nearly triples her risk of becoming obese herself. Weight gain likely spreads through friends via a process of shifting norms. If our gang meets at a fast-food restaurant every Friday night, we'll begin to believe this is normal behavior, whereas another group in the same town might consider this taboo. Just spending time with your friends can reduce your stress levels. Specifically, women felt less anxious as the result of a progesterone surge that comes on when they feel close to a friend.

Laughing with friends can increase physical pain thresholds by about 10%, and having a friend with you, or even merely imagining a friend, causes drops in blood pressure. Elderly people with active social lives are much less likely to experience cognitive decline and dementia. A more recent study confirms the inverse of this finding: Older people's dementia risk increases with their feelings of loneliness.

In one striking study, breast cancer patients who were socially isolated had a full 66% increased risk of dying compared to women with a supportive circle. It may not be because friends physiologically treat cancer so much as because they help the patient stay hopeful, attentive and compliant with the treatment at hand.

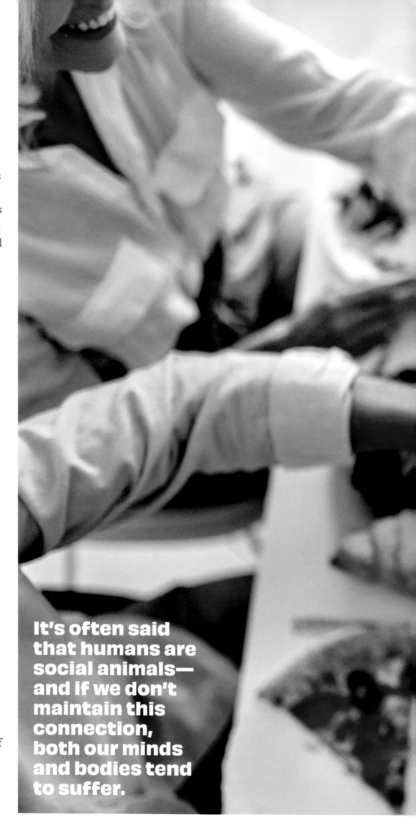

itself into what's called the "default network." The default network, when looked at through brain-imaging technology, happens to match what our brains do when we're trying to figure out other people and our relationships with them. Lieberman thinks this means we evolved to ponder social life in our free time because it is a valuable pursuit—one central to our survival.

Lieberman's lab has found that the brain's reward system lights up when we give to others and when we comfort loved ones in pain. Social rejection, in fact, is processed in the same brain region as is physical pain.

Throughout life, social connections serve as buffers against stress, which, in its chronic form, is associated with depression, anxiety and autoimmune disorders, among other afflictions. As maddening as relationships can be, not having any is far worse than having conflicts or complaints about our loved ones.

Social neuroscientist John Cacioppo of the University of Chicago describes loneliness as the fallout of not fulfilling a biological need for social contact, a need that's almost as strong as thirst or hunger. Thanks to his work, we know that loneliness is associated with the progression of disease, alcoholism and suicidal ideation. Chronic loneliness, he's shown, is associated with depression, cardiovascular

It's often said that humans are social animals—and if we don't maintain this connection, both our minds and bodies tend to suffer.

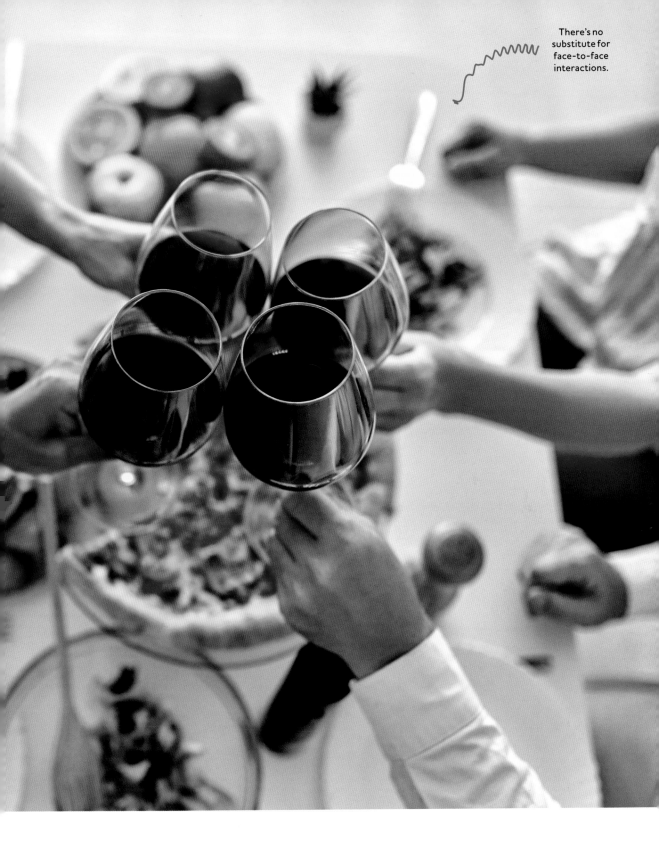

There's no substitute for face-to-face interactions.

Social Media and the Brain

STAYING CONNECTED TO OTHERS HAS ITS BENEFITS—BUT BEING ON SOCIAL MEDIA TOO MUCH CAN BACKFIRE.

Aliens landing on Earth would instantly note our obsession with screens, which has dramatically changed the way we socialize. Social networking accounts for 28% of all media time spent online, and people between ages 15 and 19 spend at least three hours a day, on average, on Facebook, Twitter and Instagram.

Surprisingly, a Nielsen report concluded that millennials ages 18 to 34 are a bit less into social media than Gen-Xers ages 35 to 49. The former group is on social media networks around six hours a week compared to the latter's seven hours. Adults 50 and over clocked about four hours.

It would be naive to think all this scrolling isn't affecting our brains and mental health. Some studies suggest that the more we use Facebook, the less happy we are; others correlate social media use with satisfaction and civic engagement.

Though we've plenty to be concerned about,

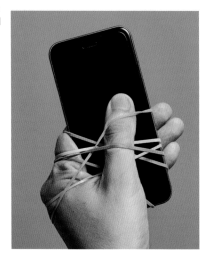

sociologist Keith Hampton of Rutgers University in New Jersey says the dangers are mostly exaggerated. Fear of new technologies characterizes sociology. "From electricity to the telephone, sociologists have argued that advances cause a decline in family and community life," he says. "These arguments have kept social scientists in business for years."

We know that social media has apparently made friendships more persistent (we no longer give up most ties as we move into new phases of life) and more pervasive (we have 24-hour access to information about people we know). "The criticism is that these tidbits are meaningless," says Hampton. "But maybe the fluff accumulates into something substantive."

Psychologist Larry Rosen, author of *iDisorder*, agrees social media is stimulating, but says too much can feed into insomnia, anxiety or depression. Evidence concurs: One team found that teens diagnosed with Internet Addiction Disorder had impaired white matter fibers in brain regions involving emotion, decision-making and cognitive control. Psychologist Andrea Bonior says the No. 1 casualty of excessive online use is time that could be better spent doing something like going to a park or brunch with friends.

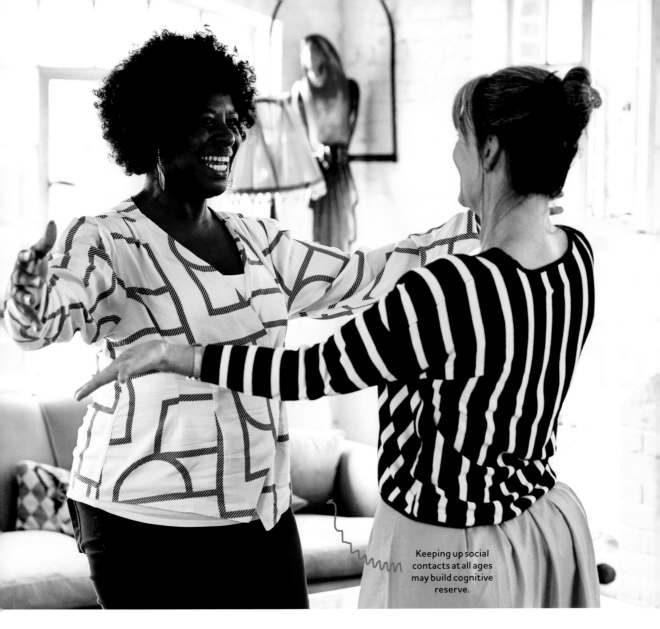

Keeping up social contacts at all ages may build cognitive reserve.

problems, sleep dysfunction, high blood pressure and an increased risk of dementia in older age.

Last year, Kay Tye and her colleagues from MIT pinpointed a region of the brain that they think generates the feeling of loneliness; some of us suffer more from that feeling than others. But in the end, you have to go out into the world to combat feelings of isolation, even if that requires taking risks. Those who are intimidated by the notion of making friends are not alone in their loneliness, as it turns out. The solution for them is to redouble their efforts to make friends, despite the discomfort it brings. Indeed, in a study published in the *Journal of Clinical Child & Adolescent Psychology* in 2016, Cacioppo reported that the best antidote for teens with a greater inner feeling of loneliness was simply to spend more time in the company of intimate others. The ability to make friends is like a muscle, and the more we exercise it, the stronger it—and we—will be.

THE POWER OF Sleep

* EVERY NIGHT, THE SLEEPING BRAIN CONSOLIDATES NEW MEMORIES AND PREPARES ITSELF FOR DAILY EMOTIONAL AND COGNITIVE CONTROL.

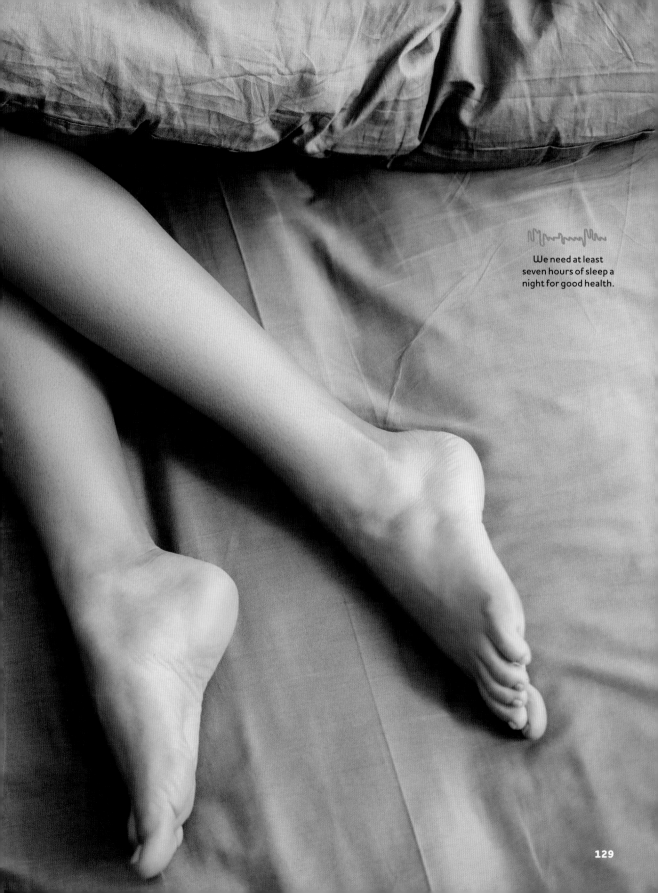

We need at least seven hours of sleep a night for good health.

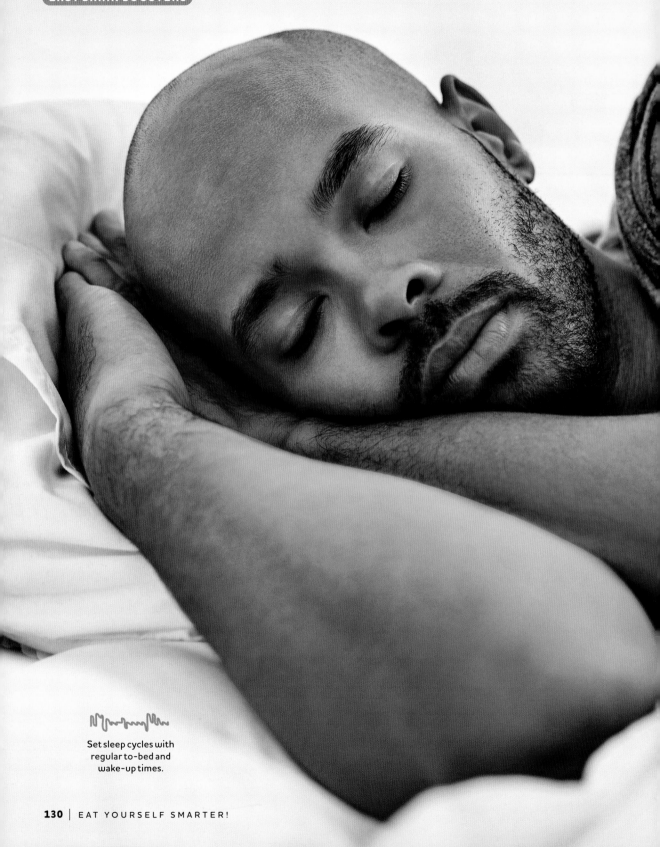

Set sleep cycles with
regular to-bed and
wake-up times.

Everyone has skimped on sleep now and then, and the outcome is never good. Lack of sleep not only triggers fatigue, it results in whole-body pain and fuzzy thinking, including loss of cognitive sharpness and emotional control. With our caffeinated lives, our lit-up cities and our 24-7 immersion in email and texts, the problem has become epidemic: The Centers for Disease Control and Prevention (CDC) reports that a third of Americans are chronically sleep-deprived. In addition to raising the risk for diabetes, obesity and heart disease, sleep loss can cause mood swings, depression and memory problems. And by disrupting the body's master control center—the brain—lack of sleep slows reaction time, a deficit that can kill on the road.

EMOTIONS AND SLEEP

Much about sleep remains a mystery, but scientists are slowly unraveling why lack of it undermines our function when we're awake. One set of studies, from Tel Aviv University in Israel, documents the emotional reactivity that emerges when too much sleep is lost. To investigate the impaired emotional control that famously follows sleep loss, the researchers asked 18 sleep-deprived participants to press buttons while viewing pictures that, in most people, spark negativity (a mutilated body), neutrality (a spoon) or positivity (a pet cat). After a night of adequate sleep, participants repeated the test, and during both trials they were monitored with MRI to document blood flow and oxygenation to areas of the brain as well as EEGs, which recorded electrical brain activity. The result? Well-rested research subjects were only distracted by the negative image, but when volunteers were sleep-deprived, they were distracted by every picture put in front of them—positive, negative or neutral.

"These results reveal that, without sleep, the mere recognition of what is an emotional and what is a neutral event is disrupted," said neuroscientist Talma Hendler, founding director of the Tel Aviv Center for Brain Function. "We may experience similar emotional provocations from all incoming events, even neutral ones, and lose our ability to sort out more or less important information."

DEEP SLEEP AND LEARNING

Sleep medicine expert Aneesa Das of Ohio State University frequently counsels students not to stay up all night to study. "It can backfire," she says, "and affect performance on exams."

Whether you are a student or not, getting enough deep sleep is key to optimal learning and remembering. Your brain cycles through several stages of sleep, starting with light sleep when brain waves start to slow from their daytime alertness patterns. Next, you enter REM (rapid eye movement) sleep, where your brain is active and you dream. Scientists believe it's during this time that the brain processes what happened during the day, including what you've learned.

After an hour or two, you snooze your way into a period of deep, non-REM sleep. Your heartbeat, breathing and brain waves slow to their lowest levels during this phase of sleep, which has to last long enough that your brain and body can be refreshed.

Lack of sleep can impact memory, cognition, mood and quality of life, especially if it turns into a chronic problem.

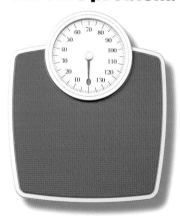

If this phase is too short or disturbed, memory can suffer, too.

In one series of experiments, Swiss researchers had volunteers learn a series of tapping exercises during the day. At night, they slept undisturbed, with their brain's electrical activity monitored by EEG to show they had plenty of deep sleep. The next day participants were able to accurately perform the exercises they had learned.

Then the experiment was repeated, but this time the scientists pulsed sound waves during the deepest part of sleep. Although the volunteers stayed asleep, their ability to remember the finger exercises the next day fell precipitously.

In real life, deep sleep can be interrupted unbeknownst to you as well: the TV might be left on, a dog outside might start to bark or you might have sleep apnea, which is marked by shallow breaths. Most people with sleep apnea don't realize this is happening but end up with excessive sleepiness and impaired memory and focus during the day.

PRUNING THE BRAIN, EMPTYING THE TRASH

It's not rocket science to recognize that sleep deprivation at night can damage your memory and ability to concentrate the next day. But it *is* brain science to figure out why this is true. The brain must recuperate from

Sleep allows the brain to reset, helping integrate newly learned material with existing memories so the brain can begin anew the next day.

functioning at full speed during the day when you are awake and neurons are constantly firing. University of Wisconsin-Madison neuroscientist Giulio Tononi believes that's the ultimate purpose of sleep.

Synapses are gaps at the end of brain cells that link neurons, allowing them to communicate. According to Tononi's theory, an enormous number of these synaptic connections are made and strengthened during the day, saturating the brain with new information. But this strengthening of synapses is a major source of cellular stress, and it can't go on without a break. So the excess synaptic connections need to be pruned down—and that's what sleep does.

Sleep allows the brain to reset, helping integrate newly learned material with existing memories so that the brain can begin anew the next day, Tononi explains.

Tononi and his colleagues have evidence from animal experiments, published in

Science, to back up their idea that the brain prunes itself during sleep. Brain tissue from mice sleeping normally was compared to samples from other mice kept awake for long periods. The researchers found the size and shape of thousands of synapses were almost 20% smaller in the mice that had been allowed to sleep compared to those in the rest-deprived rodents.

There's additional evidence that your brain uses sleep as a do-it-yourself cleanup system from neurologist Maiken Nedergaard, co-director of the Center for Translational Neuromedicine at the University of Rochester Medical Center.

Research by Nedergaard and colleagues has revealed the brain has something akin to a trash-removal service that becomes highly active during sleep. Neurons shrink, allowing waste to be removed more effectively through a process Nedergaard and colleagues have discovered and dubbed the glymphatic system. They believe this system drives cerebrospinal fluid to flow through spaces around brain cells during sleep, purging unwanted proteins and other wastes into the circulatory system and eventually out of the body.

"The difference is when we are awake, the brain cells are working very hard at processing all the information about our surroundings whereas during sleep, [they work] very, very hard

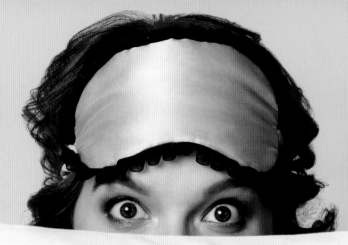

Warning! You may not be getting all the Z's you need.

Are You Sleep-Deprived?

Do you fall asleep as soon as your head hits the pillow? Do you need an alarm clock to wake up? If so, you are sleepier than you think, according to James Maas, a pioneer of sleep research while at Cornell University and co-author with Rebecca Robbins of *Sleep for Success!* To find out whether you need more sleep, determine how many of these red flags are true for you. If you say yes to at least four statements, attend to your sleep hygiene.

* Weekday mornings I often hit the snooze bar several times.

* I feel tired and stressed during the week.

* I often feel slow with critical thinking.

* I need caffeine to make it through the afternoon.

* I often wake up craving junk food and sugars.

* I tend to fall asleep watching TV.

* I fall asleep in lectures or after heavy meals.

* I need an alarm clock to get out of bed.

to remove all the wastes that build up when we are awake," Nedergaard explains.

"Our study, I believe, pinpointed that sleep is absolutely essential for the removal of toxic waste products from the active brain. The glymphatic system functions very much like a garbage-removal system," she adds.

Nedergaard's ongoing research suggests an accumulation of wastes that aren't flushed out of the body explains why a lack of enough sleep, or sleep that's not restful enough, is known to mess up memory and the ability to learn—and likely plays a role in the development of Alzheimer's and other neurodegenerative diseases.

Indeed, the connection between sleep and Alzheimer's has been made by neuroscientist Matthew Walker, director of University of California, Berkeley, Center for Human Sleep Science. To do their work, Walker and his team enrolled 26 older adults, all free of diagnosed dementia or other neurodegenerative, sleep or psychiatric disorders. The volunteers first had PET scans to measure beta-amyloid plaques, associated with Alzheimer's, in their brains. Then they were instructed to memorize 120 pairs of words and tested to see how well they remembered half of the word pairs.

After sleeping for eight hours, the research subjects were tested again to see how

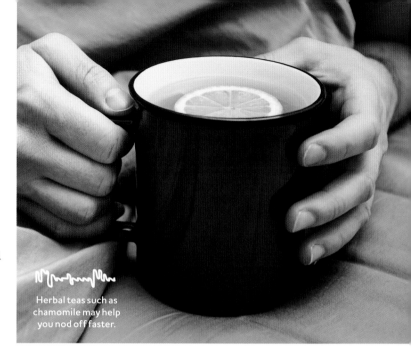

Herbal teas such as chamomile may help you nod off faster.

many of the remaining word pairs they remembered. While they worked on the memory exam, MRIs tracked activity in their hippocampus, the part of the brain where memories are temporarily stored before moving to permanent memory banks in the prefrontal cortex.

The results of the study, published in *Nature Neuroscience,* revealed that the elders with the highest levels of beta-amyloid had the poorest quality of sleep. In addition, they also scored the worst on the memory test the second day. Some had forgotten about half the word pairs they originally had memorized.

Not surprisingly, brain scans showed abnormal memory consolidation in the hippocampus. But which condition came first—lack of sleep or the damaging plaque?

"The more beta-amyloid you have in certain parts of your

brain, the less deep sleep you get and, consequently, the worse your memory," Walker explains. "Additionally, the less deep sleep you have, the less effective you are at clearing out this bad protein. It's a vicious cycle. But we don't yet know which of these two factors—the bad sleep or the bad protein—launches the cascade."

The UC Berkeley team concluded that insufficient or poor-quality sleep is an important risk factor in the memory decline of Alzheimer's. And whatever role sleep plays in the development of this devastating brain disease, they believe adequate, deep sleep could potentially offer preventative and treatment benefits.

"This discovery offers hope," Walker says. "Sleep could be a novel therapeutic target for fighting back against memory impairment in older adults."

FIVE LITTLE-KNOWN WAYS TO IMPROVE SLEEP

THERE ARE PLENTY OF WELL-KNOWN DO'S AND DON'TS FOR IMPROVING YOUR SLEEP, SUCH AS AVOIDING CAFFEINE LATE IN THE DAY AND MAKING SURE YOUR BED IS COMFORTABLE AND YOUR ROOM IS COOL. BUT IF STANDARD TACTICS AREN'T WORKING AND YOU HAVE DIFFICULTY FALLING AND STAYING ASLEEP— OR YOU FREQUENTLY WAKE UP TIRED AND UNREFRESHED—CONSIDER THESE OFTEN-OVERLOOKED STRATEGIES TO SOOTHE AND IMPROVE YOUR SLUMBER TIME.

1 **LIMIT ALCOHOL** Drinking a glass of wine can help you fall asleep, but booze may also cause you to wake up one or two hours later, explains Emory University sleep disorders specialist David Schulman. "For better sleep, don't drink a couple of hours before you go to bed."

2 **AVOID CARBS** If you tend to get heartburn or suffer from gastroesophageal reflux disease (GERD), eating close to bedtime can make symptoms worse and disrupt sleep. For other people who crave a nighttime snack, Schulman advises avoiding leftover pizza, cookies and other high-carb foods and opting for a small protein-rich snack, such as cheese, milk or lean meat. "We think carbs affect blood sugar levels and can cause significant sleep disruption," Schulman states.

3 **KEEP YOUR BEDROOM DARK** Exposure to light suppresses the secretion of melatonin, a sleep-promoting hormone that influences your circadian rhythm (a kind of internal clock). Any light can disrupt sleep, but it's especially important to shut down your computer, tablet and phone because they emit short-wavelength blue light, which impacts melatonin levels more strongly than other light sources, disrupting sleep cycles and causing early morning grogginess.

4 **RESTRICT EXERCISE** When you have trouble relaxing at the end of a busy day, exercise can help— but doesn't always promote sleep. A workout too late in the evening can rev you up instead of making you sleepy. "Those fight-or-flight hormones stick around and can make it harder to fall asleep," Schulman explains.

5 **MASTER MINDFULNESS** Schulman recommends relaxation techniques, including yoga and meditation, for reducing stress. He also believes in cognitive behavioral therapy (CBT), a form of talk therapy, to help you control thoughts and emotions that can stop you getting adequate sleep, though mastery can take weeks or months. If all these strategies fail, talk to your doctor, Schulman adds. Get to the bottom of your sleep problem without taking sleeping pills, which could mask a problem you need to fix.

Avoid the nightcap— it can backfire.

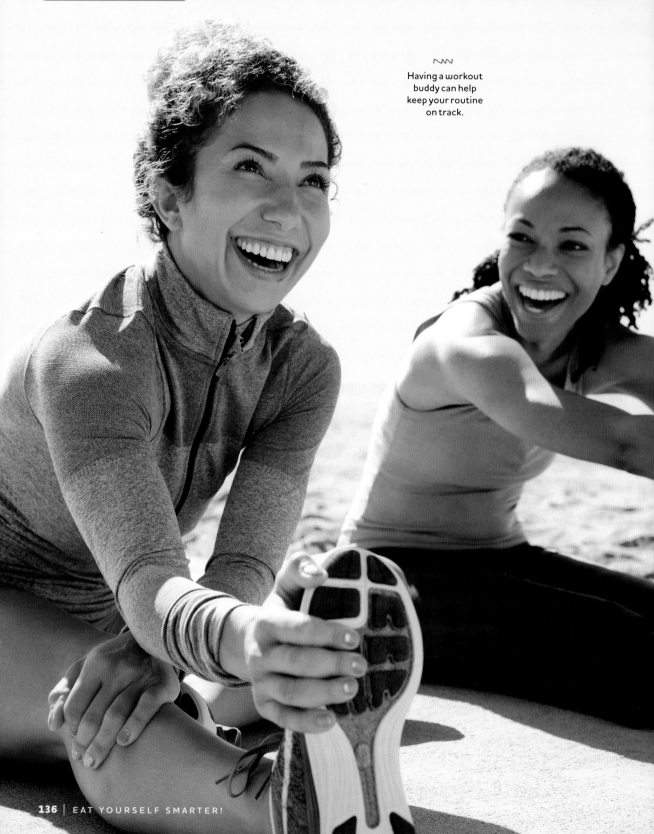

Having a workout buddy can help keep your routine on track.

YOUR BRAIN on EXERCISE

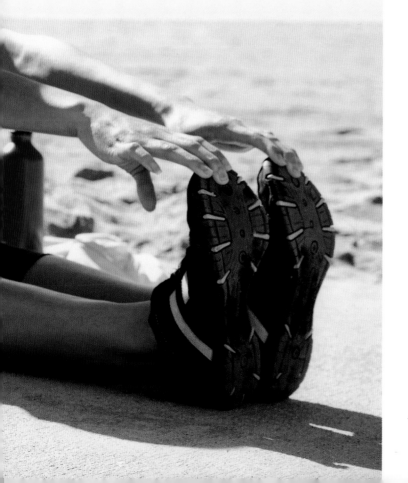

*

AEROBICS, YOGA AND EVEN DANCE CAN REDUCE DEPRESSION, STOP YOU FROM RUMINATING AND INCREASE YOUR ABILITY TO FOCUS AT WORK.

It might be time to put aside those crossword puzzles and lace up your sneakers instead: "The most important thing that any of us can do to protect our brain from aging and improve brain function is physical exercise," says geriatric psychiatrist Gary Small, director of the UCLA Longevity Center. "Many people think of exercise as something that helps your muscles and stamina, but it also has tremendous benefits for brain health."

Most scientists long assumed that the adult brain was "hardwired." But in the 1990s, an avalanche of research concluded that the brain is indeed plastic and able to adapt and improve throughout our lives, says Wendy Suzuki, a neuroscientist at New York University.

"When you exercise, you're getting your heart to pump faster, you're getting nutrients and oxygen to your brain cells, and your body is producing chemicals such as BDNF—brain-derived

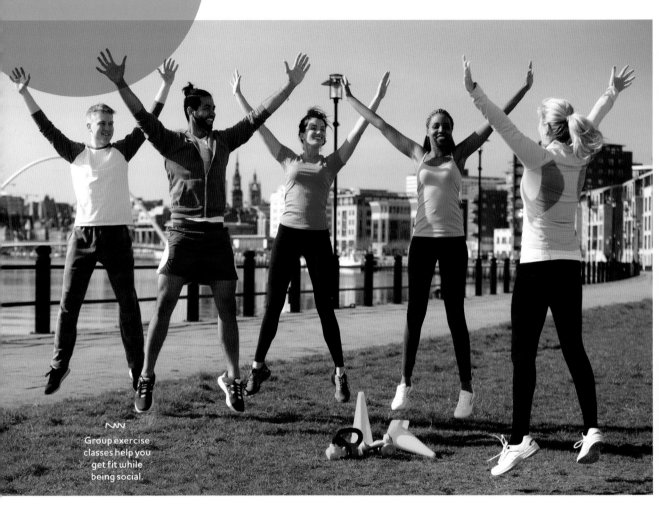

Group exercise classes help you get fit while being social.

neurotrophic factor—which is like fertilizer for your brain," says Small. "It gets your neurons to sprout branches, so your cells communicate better."

Exercise not only strengthens the bonds between nerve cells, it also spurs the genesis of new nerve cells. Whereas new cells can only form in the hippocampus (a memory center) and olfactory bulb (the smell center), connections between

cells can be formed and enhanced all over the brain.

For example, a 2011 study showed that older adults who engaged in moderate-intensity aerobic exercise (which includes brisk walking) just 45 minutes a day, three days a week, for a year had more volume in their hippocampus areas. The exercise literally reversed the normal loss of volume in the hippocampus that occurs with age, damaging

memory and increasing risk of dementia. It's an important finding, since one new case of dementia is detected every four seconds around the world. Greater hippocampal volume was linked to improvement of spatial memory as well.

Exercise can keep you on task, too. One study of children found that exercising for 20 minutes between lessons improved their attention spans. There's

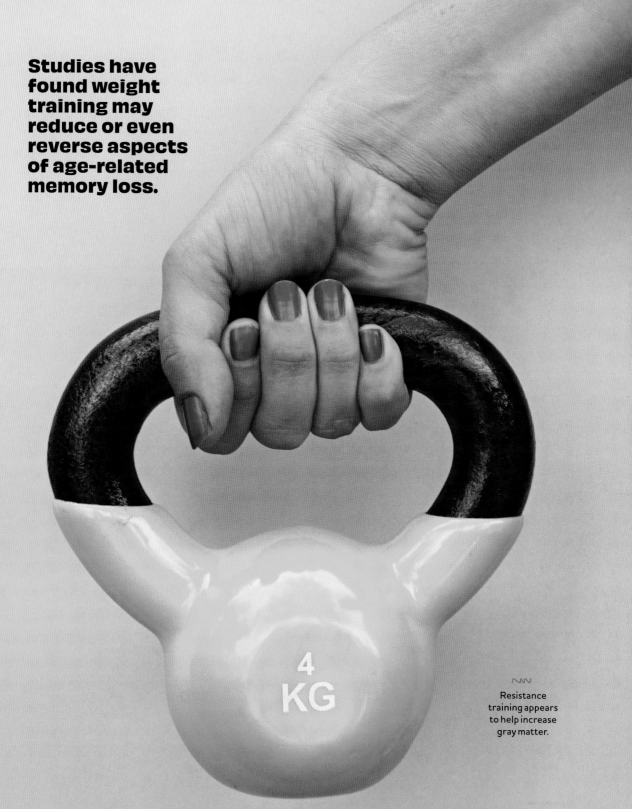

Studies have found weight training may reduce or even reverse aspects of age-related memory loss.

Resistance training appears to help increase gray matter.

4 KG

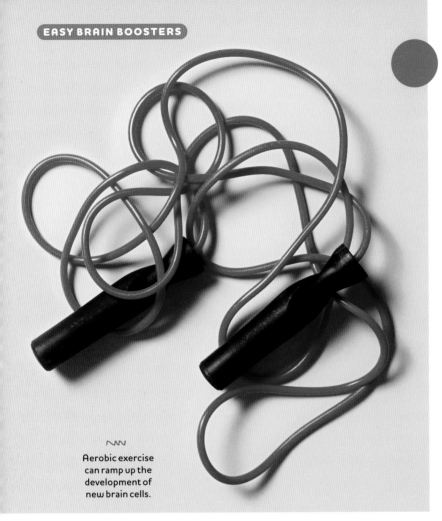

Aerobic exercise can ramp up the development of new brain cells.

and widely documented. "If you don't exercise, then hormones that increase with stress will tend to damage brain cells and make them shrink," Suzuki says. "By contrast, in a brain that has experienced exercise, that same stressor will have no effect because there are more growth factors in the brain that help protect it from the negative effects of stress."

MOOD-BOOSTING MOVES

Exercise has a strong effect on psychological as well as cognitive health. Exciting news comes from a recent meta-analysis (analysis of many studies in aggregate) involving a million subjects in all. Conducted by exercise physiologist Felipe Schuch from the Centro Universitário La Salle in Brazil, the massive analysis confirms that aerobic exercise can prevent depression. People with low cardiorespiratory fitness had a 75% higher risk of developing depression later on, while people with medium fitness levels had a 23% higher risk.

"Depression is a hard-to-treat disorder, and exercise can be added to pharmacological therapies and psychotherapies," Schuch says. "Sometimes, starting to exercise is the harder step, so antidepressants can provide that initial motivation."

"Exercise is activating nearly all of your body's systems, so to think we'll be able to pinpoint one

also evidence that kids who participate in sports every day have superior executive control, meaning that they can better handle information, multitask and deal with distractions.

A dash to the gym might even help you be more creative back at the office: A set of experiments conducted in 2014 demonstrated that after walking on a treadmill, adults scored better on tests of creative divergent thinking. Walking outdoors produced even better results, which is not surprising, since nature's positive effects on mental

functioning are powerful and well known.

Exercise also reduces inflammation, which is part of the body's stress response system. Inflammation in the brain has been linked to compromised thinking, not to mention neurodegenerative disease. Keeping inflammation down is a prerequisite for physical and mental health.

Finally, people who exercise tend to sleep better and feel less stress. The effects of chronic stress and lack of sleep on cognitive function are deep

Five Ways to Cross-Train Your Brain

HOW MUCH EXERCISE—AND WHAT KINDS—DO YOU NEED TO ENHANCE YOUR BRAIN? THERE'S NO SINGLE ANSWER, BUT THERE ARE A VARIETY OF PROSPECTIVE ACTIVITIES (AND INTENSITIES) TO CHOOSE FROM.

1 **COMBINE AEROBICS AND MEDITATION** to fight depression and reduce rumination. "In the literature of exercise, if you want to see a reduction in depression, we would say you'd have to exercise for a minimum of 10 weeks, three times a week, for about 30 to 45 minutes each session," Brandon Alderman says. In his study of meditation and exercise, subjects meditated for just 30 minutes, followed by a 30-minute session of aerobic exercise, twice a week for eight weeks. "Though it was a lower dose of exercise, the overall affect size of that trial was much larger than what we see across the literature. This suggests that there is something unique about combining exercise and meditation," says Alderman.

2 **MEDITATION PLUS YOGA** can lift your mood. Volunteers who did yoga and meditation for 12 weeks showed more improvements in their mood and less of a risk of depression than subjects in a "brain-training" group that performed mental exercises. The yoga group also had better visuospatial memories, which helps with navigation, and a greater ability to focus.

3 **DANCE AGAINST DEMENTIA** A study of elderly subjects found that dancing regularly, much more so than 11 other types of physical activities, warded off dementia. In addition to being a mood-booster, dance is a unique form of exercise. "Dancing engages emotions, the motor system, the cognitive system, and it is highly social. It is a remarkably comprehensive brain-enriching activity," explains Ian Robertson, a neuroscientist at the Center for BrainHealth at the University of Texas at Dallas.

4 **A FEW MINUTES OF YOGA** can lower inflammation and boost immunity. A study of stressed-out caregivers showed that practicing a mere 12 minutes of yoga every day for eight weeks reduced the inflammation response in the brain. It also boosted antiviral response to levels seen in less stressed-out groups.

5 **WORK OUT WITH FRIENDS** Try exercising with others to achieve the sense of social connection that improves cognitive function, including attention and alertness, along with mood. Working out in a group also increases our motivation to stick with the program, so recruit your friends as you train your brain.

mechanism for how it impacts depression is a bit naive," adds Brandon Alderman, director of the Exercise Psychophysiology Lab at Rutgers University. He has studied the impairments in cognitive function that often accompany depression, such as ruminating on worries. Aerobic exercise reduces rumination, and Alderman found that combining running with meditation is particularly helpful in combating the symptoms of depression.

Suzuki is trying to figure out what everyone wants to know: How much do you have to exercise to improve your brain? "We still don't have the exact prescription," she says, "but you can improve your mood just by going for a walk—you don't even have to break a sweat."

One of her studies looked at the immediate effects of just one bout of aerobic exercise and found it leads to improved attention and mood and decreased stress levels. It could be that exercise produces proteins (such as BDNF) that improve the covering on synapses that makes the messages sent from one neuron to another travel faster.

Runners might also have an edge on other exercisers in terms of sprouting new brain cells: A study with rats compared the effects of running versus resistance training (yes, tiny weights were affixed to the rodents' tails) versus high-intensity

Exercise spikes levels of feel-good chemicals in the brain.

Physical activity guidelines recommend most adults get at least 150 minutes of moderate exercise a week.

interval training (HIIT) on the brain. After seven weeks, the jogging rats had many more new cells in their hippocampal tissue, which correlated with the distance each rat had run during the study. (Rats that tried high-intensity interval training had far fewer new neurons, and the weight trainers didn't have any.)

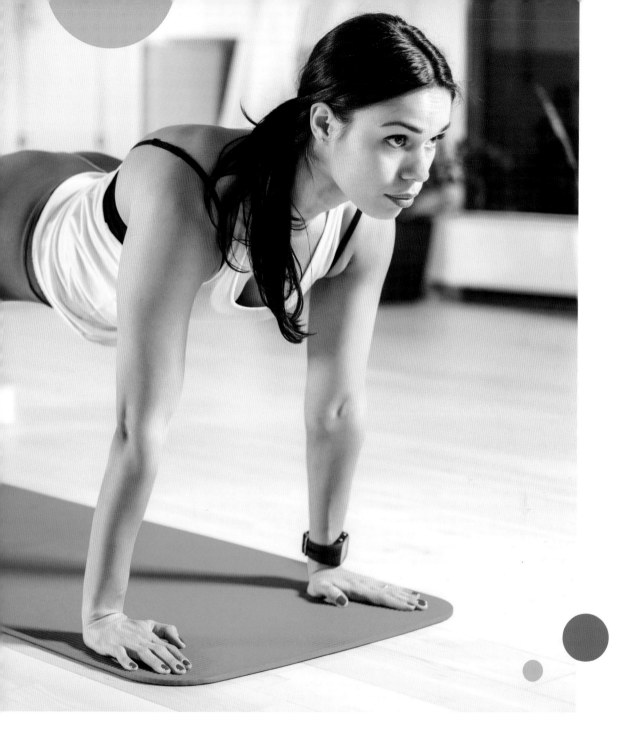

But strength training appears to have its own bonuses for the brain beyond the direct impact of exercise itself: "If you have more lean muscle mass, your muscles burn more calories. So it's easier to reach your ideal body weight, and we know that obesity and being overweight is not good for cognitive health," says Small. Since our bodies and minds are closely intertwined, any kind of exercise that helps our bodies is bound to be good for our brains in some way.

THE MAGIC OF
Meditation

You love how you feel after meditation. But have you ever wondered what it does to you—specifically to your brain? It's a hot area of research, and thanks to devices like magnetic resonance imaging (MRI) machines, scientists are now able to track what goes on in your head and what effect meditation may have on your mind.

While research is still in the preliminary stages (brains are a tough nut to crack), the findings are eye-opening: In addition to calming your heart rate and relaxing your muscles, meditation appears to affect the brain in ways that can last far beyond your time on the cushion. It may be useful in boosting concentration and attention, and offer new help for people combating addiction and depression. It may even alter the structure of the brain itself, making desirable areas, such as ones that control memory, more dense, while shrinking parts that control negative emotions.

"I see this area of focus continuing to move in a positive direction as we begin to get real, meaningful results from our studies, and as many people move their health-care focus to preventative medicine and away from a purely pharmacological approach," says Robert Kaufman, a lab manager and clinical research coordinator at the Lazar Laboratory in Boston, which is affiliated with Massachusetts General Hospital. Might you eventually get a script from your doctor to meditate as treatment for your anxiety or high blood pressure? "The research is not quite to that level yet, but we already see some clinical psychologists using meditation as a part of treatment for their patients suffering from things like anxiety and depression," Kaufman says.

As studies ramp up around the world, we asked some leading meditation researchers, here and abroad, to share the details of their work. Read on to learn how they conduct their investigations, as well as some of the exciting findings in this field.

HOW THE GOOD STUFF HAPPENS

Researchers use many different techniques to study meditation, from simple questionnaires and skin tests to blood work, MRIs and EEGs (electroencephalograms). "The exact measures we take depend on the aim of the study," says Britta Hölzel, PhD, a neuroscientist with the Technical University of Munich.

Study participants are usually introduced to meditation through a class. "One that's often used for research studies is an eight-week Mindfulness-Based Stress Reduction (MBSR) course that consists of once-weekly group meetings as well as a daily homework practice," says Hölzel. "The MBSR course is used because it is a manualized, standardized training." It's set, and easy to reproduce.

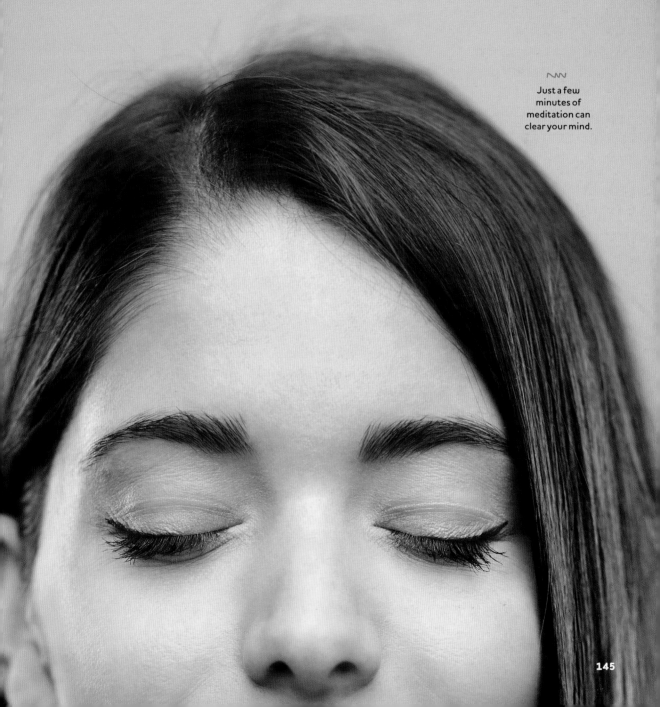

*
THE BENEFITS MAY BE BEYOND WHAT WE EVER IMAGINED—SEE WHAT SCIENTISTS ARE SAYING ABOUT HOW THIS SIMPLE ACT MAY MOLD YOUR MIND.

Just a few minutes of meditation can clear your mind.

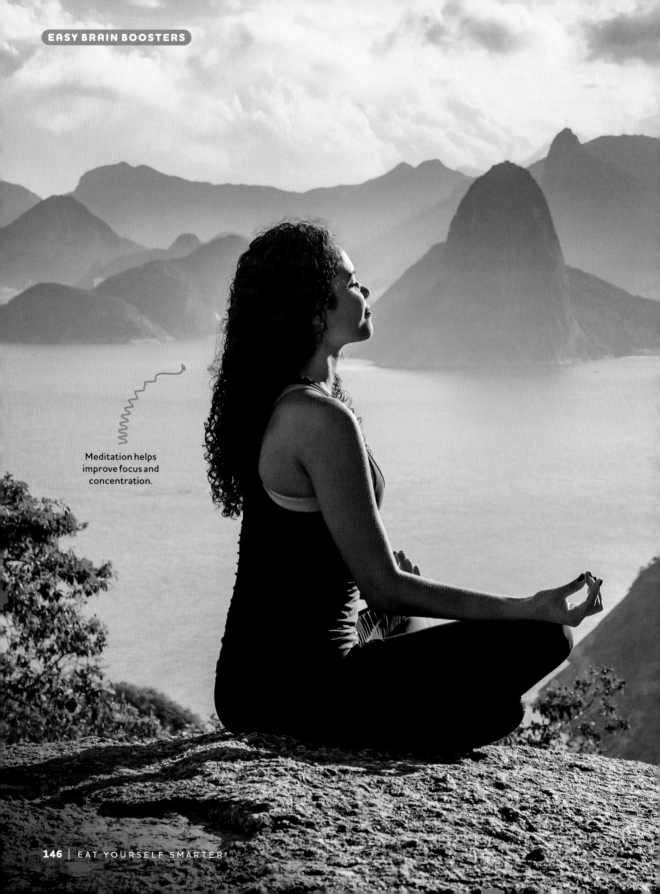

Meditation helps improve focus and concentration.

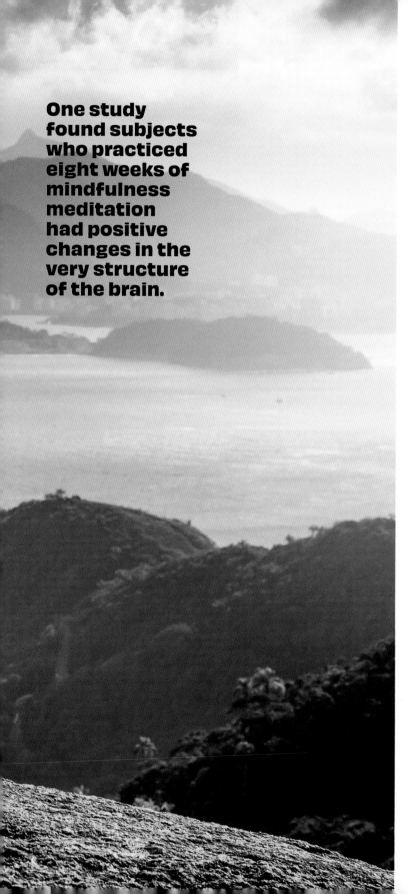

One study found subjects who practiced eight weeks of mindfulness meditation had positive changes in the very structure of the brain.

"I would say the real magic of what we do comes in the form of MRIs," says Kaufman. "They give us a ton of information and are very meaningful—they give weight to the argument that meditation can actually change the shape of the brain." MRI studies tend to focus on multiple areas of the brain. These include the prefrontal cortex ("sort of the focused-attention area," Kaufman says); the hippocampus, which is thought of as the memory area; the amygdala, a region responsible for a lot of emotional stimuli and strong negative stimuli, like fear responses; and the insula, a deep-brain area that is related to the functioning of the default mode network, or DMN. The DMN is a network of regions that are active when the brain is not focused on a task, such as when you're daydreaming. When you begin to focus on something, that activity is reduced. Essentially it's the network that controls self-referential thoughts and mind wandering. "This is sort of what we're looking at when we're researching meditation," says Kaufman. "Can we keep our minds from wandering and focus for a certain amount of time?"

WHAT WE'VE LEARNED SO FAR

"Although the field is still in its infancy, several research groups have reported changes in brain regions following mindfulness meditation practice," says Hölzel. Following are some of the most notable changes observed:

GREATER GRAY MATTER One study from UCLA discovered that devoted, long-term meditators (those who'd meditated for 20 years, on average) have better-preserved brains than non-meditators as they age. Their volume of gray matter (which processes information) throughout the brain was denser. And though they still lost some volume as they aged, they lost less overall than people who didn't practice meditation.

"Something that we're continually working toward is proving the hypothesis that the gray matter in the hippocampus [the memory area] will get more dense [with meditation]," Kaufman adds. In very general terms, the implication of that would be better memory or preserved memory, he says. (The Lazar Laboratory team found that eight weeks of MBSR increases cortical thickness in the hippocampus, a brain area that regulates learning and memory. At the same time, subjects showed decreases in the brain cell volume of their amygdalas.)

WEAKENED WANDERINGS Even something as simple as mindfulness meditation—where you return your attention to your breath whenever your mind wanders—can have profound effects. A study at Yale found this

How Sound Is Meditation Research?

STUDIES INTO MEDITATION'S BENEFITS UTILIZE CUTTING-EDGE TECHNOLOGY, YET THERE'S SOME BLOWBACK THAT THE RESEARCH ITSELF MAY BE FLAWED. HERE'S WHY THERE'S DEBATE:

POORLY FUNDED AND DESIGNED STUDIES
"Financial resources for the research are usually very limited, so many studies use small sample sizes, poor control groups or inappropriate designs. It is therefore important not to overstate the findings," says Britta Hölzel of the Technical University of Munich. Most of the results are preliminary, and despite some promising evidence, we don't know exactly what meditation does for us yet.

EVER-INCREASING COMMERCIALIZATION OF SCIENCE
Meditation researchers may have difficulty publishing a study that doesn't have interesting results (for example, a study finds that meditation doesn't help with impulsiveness). "To avoid shelving their research, scientists try to pull something, anything, out of their data in order to publish," says Joshua Grant, PhD, a researcher at the Max Planck Institute in Germany. "In the worst cases, they cheat statistically in order to publish."

HIGHLY BIASED RESEARCHERS
"The people who are studying meditation tend to be those who believe in the benefits," Grant points out. "They likely meditate themselves. So they have something to prove, to themselves and to others," which can influence results.

Still, there's room for optimism as data show promising results, says Robert Kaufman of Boston's Lazar Lab: "We're making each new study slightly stronger than the last."

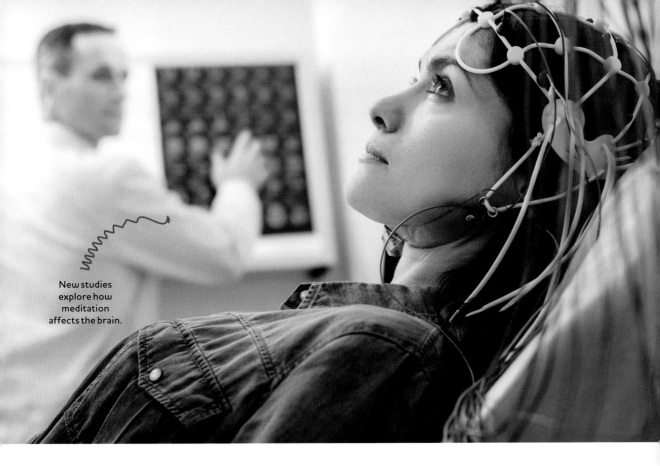

New studies explore how meditation affects the brain.

type of practice quiets activity within the DMN. That's a good thing, since mind wandering is linked to ruminating, worrying and being less happy.

IMPROVED ATTENTION AND CONCENTRATION One study found that just a few weeks of meditation training helped people focus and recall facts during the verbal reasoning section of the GRE, the test required to get into many graduate schools. Subjects experienced a boost in their average overall score (from 460 to 520) and reported fewer distracting thoughts during the test.

MORE AMMO AGAINST ADDICTION Since meditation seems to affect the brain's self-control areas, it may also help people recover from different kinds of addiction. One study found that mindfulness training was more effective than the Freedom From Smoking plan promoted by the American Lung Association. Subjects were more likely to have quit smoking by the end of training, and to continue abstaining at the 17-week follow-up point.

A LESS-ACTIVATED AMYGDALA Researcher Gaëlle Desbordes, PhD, an instructor in radiology at Harvard Medical School and a neuroscientist at Massachusetts General Hospital's Martinos Center for Biomedical Imaging, has been studying meditation's effects on the brains of clinically

depressed patients using functional MRIs. Her research has shown that after eight weeks of training in mindful attention meditation, their amygdalas are less activated. (She's also found that changes in brain activity in subjects who've learned meditation hold steady even when they're not meditating.)

"The brain changes with many things that we do," says Hölzel. "But it is fascinating that it has this enormous capacity for adaptation and that in part, we can choose where we'd like to take these processes. The skills, attitudes and capacities that we choose to cultivate shape who we are—down to the level of our brain."

Feed Your Spirit

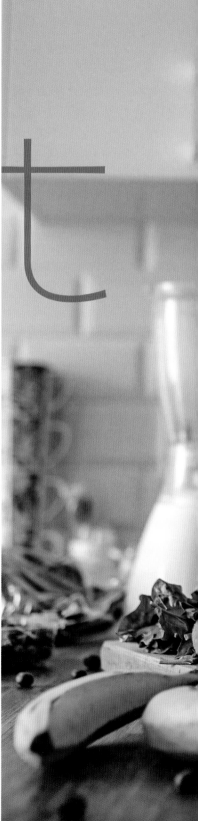

* **MINDFUL EATING MAKES THE MOST OF THE NUTRIENTS YOU TAKE IN. SO AS YOU SIT DOWN TO EAT, GIVE IT SOME THOUGHT.**

An important word before you get to the delicious recipes in the following chapter: *How* you eat may be as important to your brain as *what* you eat. As we've seen, research into mindfulness has burgeoned in the past two decades, finding that practicing meditation can have profound effects on cognitive functioning. Now, researchers are beginning to focus specifically on the practice of mindful eating—being focused and in-the-moment while sitting down to a meal—and finding that your state of mind affects how your brain and body use the nutrients you're taking in.

Mindfulness has been described as cultivating the present-moment experience, observing without judgment. A review article in the journal *Nature Reviews Neuroscience* describes some of the brain benefits that result from a regular meditation practice. These include changes in brain structure, especially in the anterior cingulate cortex, the region that's associated with attention; researchers concluded that "mindfulness practice enhances attention."

Another study, published in *Scientific Reports,* looked at mindfulness while eating and found that over an eight-week

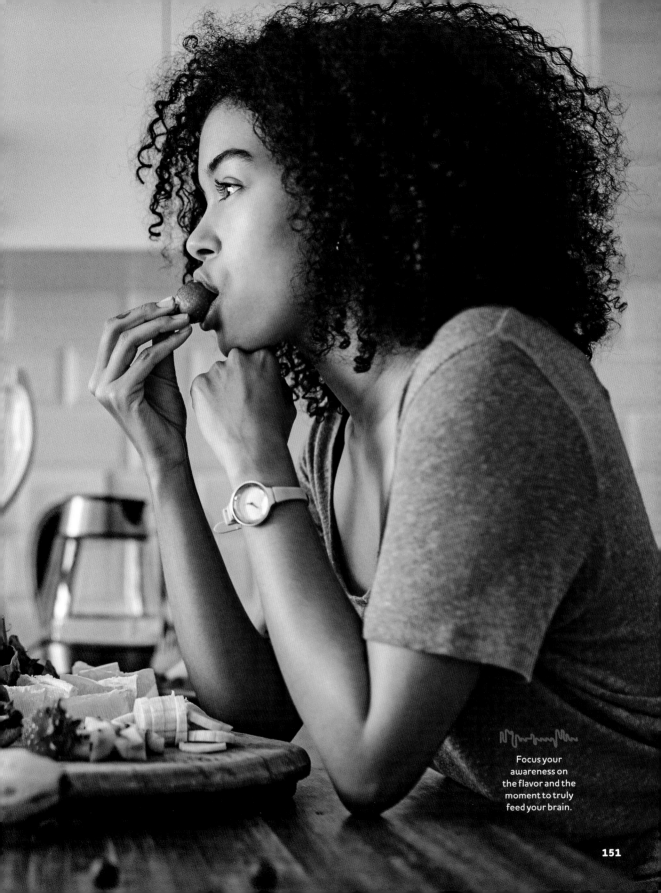

Focus your
awareness on
the flavor and the
moment to truly
feed your brain.

Taking time to
eat mindfully will
reduce digestive
discomfort.

period, practicing mindful eating changed "reward anticipation in striata and midbrain reward regions." Translation: The practice rewired participants' reward pathways that respond to food cues and cravings, short-circuiting addictive patterns that can drive people to overeat. "[This] could result in decreased food-cue triggered overeating in the long term," researchers concluded, which "might be relevant in other compulsive behaviors, such as addiction."

FOCUS ON YOUR FOOD

So mindful eating may improve your ability to focus, as well as help you break unhealthy eating patterns—but can it actually affect, and even enhance, the use of nutrients in your body? Yes, answers Leslie Korn, PhD, MPH, a specialist in integrative medicine who practices mental health nutrition and nutritional psychology. That's because mindfulness has been shown to be a powerful way to unwind, and stress is the enemy of digestion. "In order to digest, we must be relaxed," explains Korn, the author of *Nutrition Essentials for Mental Health.* "When we're stressed, the nervous system goes into a 'fight, flight or freeze' response that impairs digestive muscle contractions, reduces the secretion of digestive enzymes and redirects blood flow away from the digestive organs."

Eating a meal is not the time to multitask. Instead, slow down and pay attention to how a food smells, looks, feels and tastes, engaging all of your senses as you dine.

The stress hormone cortisol plays a key role in this response, essentially setting up a battle over which parts of your body get blood flow. Under stress, blood rushes to your muscles, in case you need to flee, and your brain, so you can figure out your options.

While blood flowing to your brain might sound helpful, it has the opposite effect when you're eating—your system should be focused on digesting your food and directing its nutrients to all the right places.

Poor digestion "affects the neurochemicals that influence mood and well-being," says Korn. Just as your brain uses neurotransmitters, so too does your gut microbiome, often called the second brain. "And a whopping 95% of the serotonin in the body, which improves mood and the ability to digest carbohydrates, is produced in the gut." Impaired digestion of protein foods also means "their amino acids are not

available to the brain to support neurotransmitter production, directly affecting mood, sleep and cravings," she adds.

MINDFUL MEALS

All of these reactions mean that, in addition to cooking brain-boosting recipes, you should start incorporating mindfulness into your mealtimes. How to do this? Rule No. 1 is to turn off the TV, computer, tablet or other distractions. Korn gives her patients these additional pointers:

* Eat in a relaxing setting.
* Employ rituals, such as communal eating and giving thanks.
* Breathe slowly and rhythmically before eating and during the meal.
* Put your fork down between bites and let it sit for 15 to 30 seconds.
* Chew your food thoroughly, concentrating on the experience: the flavor and texture, and your body's reaction.
* Bring mindfulness to the entire eating process, including food preparation. While stirring a risotto, react to the warmth, the aroma, and also to the pleasure of being with others as you share the cooking experience. "Infusing each step of the nutritional process with a ritual or mindful process enhances relationships as well as digestion and well-being," says Korn. "This social connection is where mental health nutrition begins."

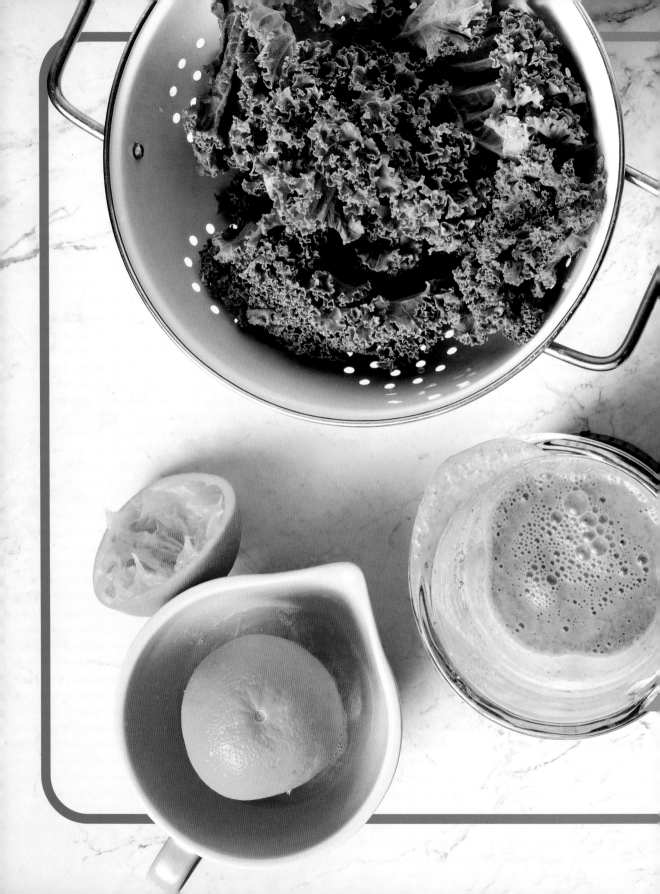

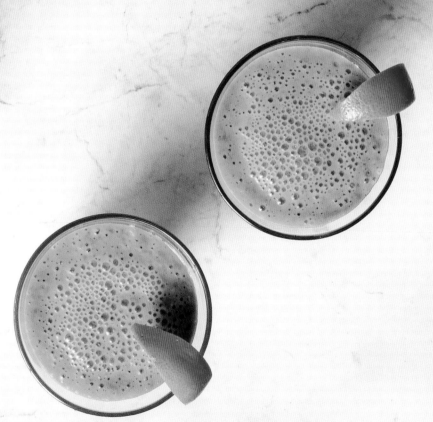

— CHAPTER 4 —

Genius

RECIPES

SMART FOOD CAN BE DELICIOUS! TRY
THESE BRAIN-HAPPY DISHES FOR MORE
MENTAL ENERGY AND BETTER MOODS.

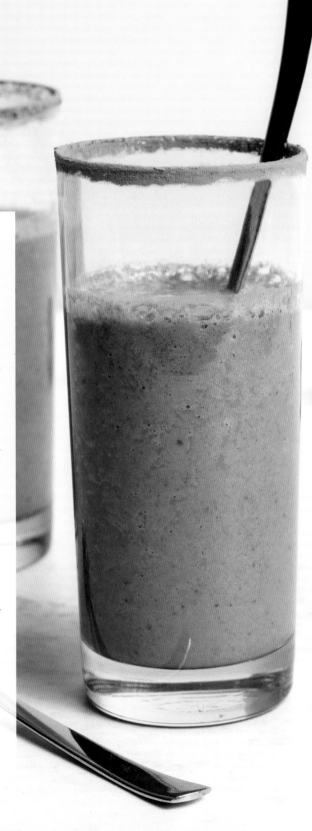

MATCHA MANGO SPINACH SMOOTHIE

Matcha—dried, powdered green tea—contains antioxidants called catechins and has been shown to improve attention and memory.

START TO FINISH 5 minutes (all active)
SERVINGS 2 (about 1 cup or 8 fluid ounces each)

INGREDIENTS

- 1 **cup unsweetened almond milk**
- 1 **teaspoon matcha powder**
- ½ **cup mango chunks**
- ½ **peeled and sliced banana**
- 1 **cup spinach leaves**
  GARNISH rim glass with matcha

INSTRUCTIONS

Place ingredients in the blender jar, in the order listed. Blend on low speed for 10 seconds, stopping to scrape down the sides of the jar with a spatula if needed. Blend on high speed for 15 seconds to fully mix. Serve immediately.

BEET ORANGE SMOOTHIE

Beets contain high levels of nitrates, which the body converts to nitric oxide to help boost blood flow to the brain. This wonderfully sweet blend will make a believer out of even the most beet-averse.

START TO FINISH 5 minutes (all active)

SERVINGS 1 (about 2 cups or 16 fluid ounces)

INGREDIENTS

$1\frac{1}{2}$ cups orange juice

1 small beet, peeled and grated

2 mandarin oranges, peeled and separated into segments

GARNISH beet slice

INSTRUCTIONS

Place ingredients in the blender jar, in the order listed. Blend on low speed for 10 seconds, stopping to scrape down the sides of the jar with a spatula if needed. Blend on high speed for 15 seconds to fully mix. Serve immediately.

Quick Tip

The same colorful antioxidant compounds that deliver beets' health benefits can stain your hands and cutting board; consider wearing disposable gloves when handling.

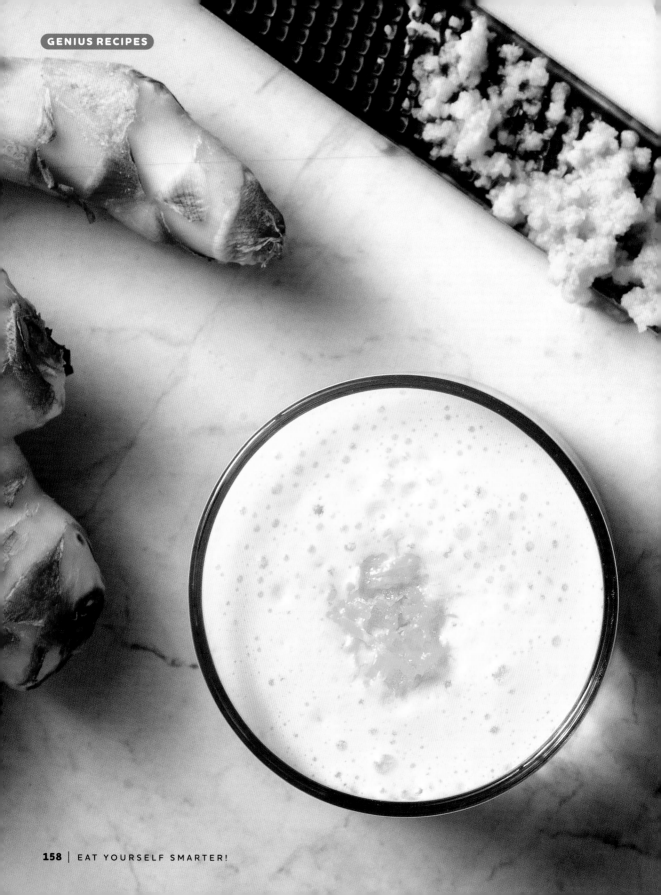

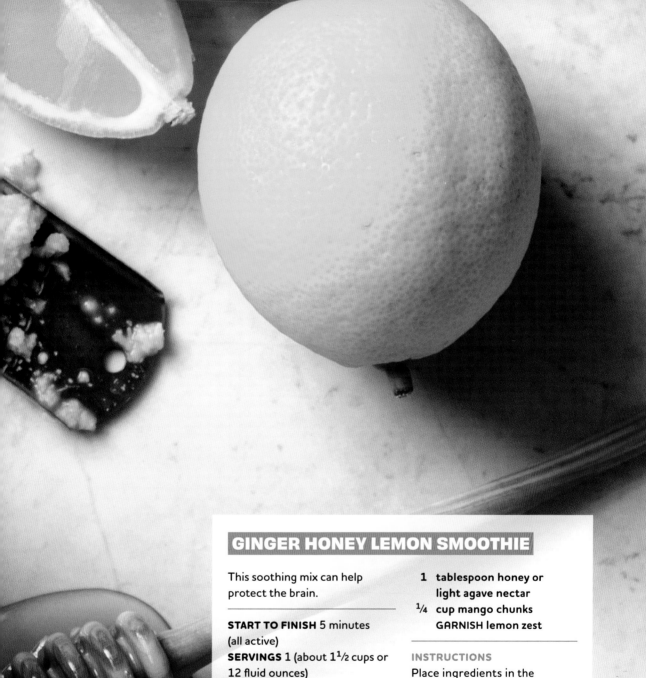

GINGER HONEY LEMON SMOOTHIE

This soothing mix can help protect the brain.

START TO FINISH 5 minutes (all active)
SERVINGS 1 (about $1^1/2$ cups or 12 fluid ounces)

INGREDIENTS

- 1 **cup unsweetened coconut milk**
  Zest and juice of half a lemon
- $1^1/2$ **tablespoons fresh grated ginger**
- 1 **tablespoon honey or light agave nectar**
- $^1/4$ **cup mango chunks**
  GARNISH lemon zest

INSTRUCTIONS

Place ingredients in the blender jar, in the order listed. Blend on low speed for 10 seconds, stopping to scrape down the sides of the jar with a spatula if needed. Blend on high speed for 15 seconds to fully mix. Serve immediately.

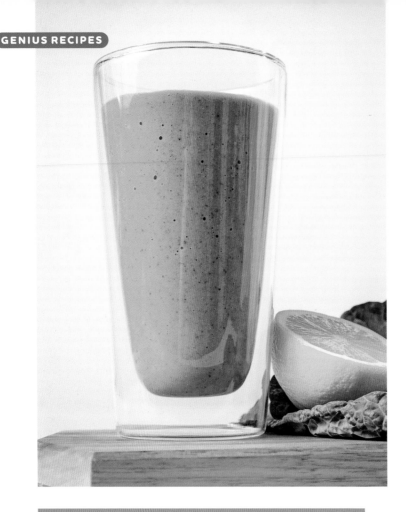

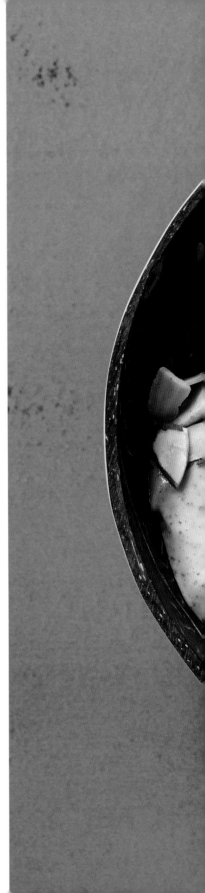

SPINACH KALE AVOCADO SMOOTHIE

Pear adds natural sweetness to this blend of greens and buttery avocado. For extra fiber, leave the skin on; for a smoother texture, remove before blending.

START TO FINISH 5 minutes (all active)
SERVINGS 1 (about 2 cups or 16 fluid ounces)

INGREDIENTS
- 1 **cup unsweetened soy milk**
- ½ **cup silken tofu**
  Squeeze of lemon juice
- 1 **teaspoon honey or light agave nectar**
- ½ **avocado, peeled and chopped**
- ½ **pear, cored, seeded and chopped**
- 1 **cup chopped lacinato or curly kale**
- 1 **cup spinach leaves**

INSTRUCTIONS
Place ingredients in the blender jar, in the order listed. Blend on low speed for 10 seconds, stopping to scrape down the sides of the jar with a spatula if needed. Blend on high speed for 15 seconds to fully mix. Serve immediately.

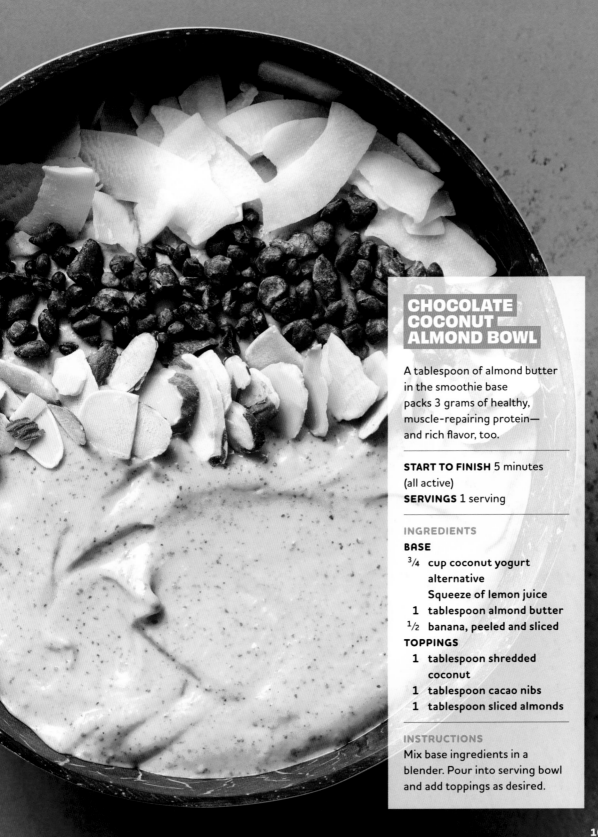

CHOCOLATE COCONUT ALMOND BOWL

A tablespoon of almond butter in the smoothie base packs 3 grams of healthy, muscle-repairing protein— and rich flavor, too.

START TO FINISH 5 minutes (all active)
SERVINGS 1 serving

INGREDIENTS
BASE
- 3/4 cup coconut yogurt alternative
- Squeeze of lemon juice
- 1 tablespoon almond butter
- 1/2 banana, peeled and sliced

TOPPINGS
- 1 tablespoon shredded coconut
- 1 tablespoon cacao nibs
- 1 tablespoon sliced almonds

INSTRUCTIONS
Mix base ingredients in a blender. Pour into serving bowl and add toppings as desired.

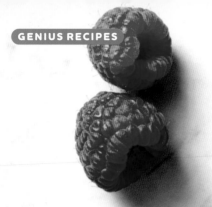

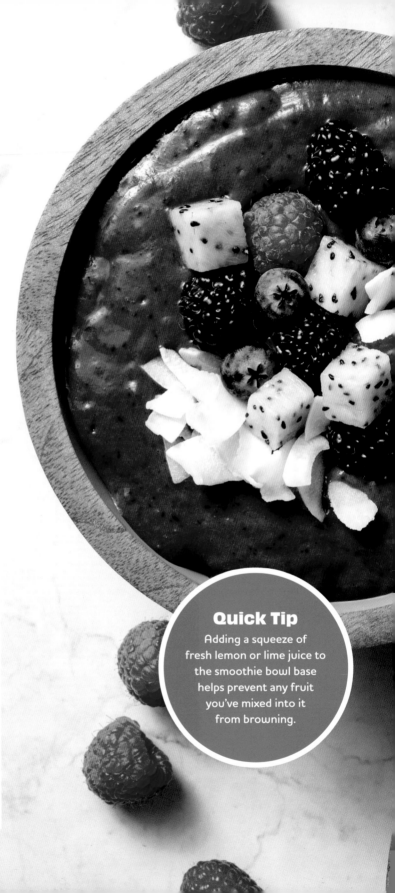

AÇAI BERRY DRAGON FRUIT BOWL

Chia seeds help this antioxidant-rich, all-fruit base gel.

START TO FINISH 5 minutes (all active)
SERVINGS 1

INGREDIENTS

BASE
- 1 (3.5-ounce) packet frozen açai pulp, slightly defrosted
- ½ cup mixed berries
- ½ peeled and sliced banana
- Squeeze of lime juice
- 1 tablespoon chia seeds

TOPPINGS
- 1 tablespoon shredded coconut
- ¼ cup mixed berries
- ¼ cup peeled and cubed dragon fruit

INSTRUCTIONS

Mix base ingredients in a blender. Pour into serving bowl and add toppings as desired.

Quick Tip

Adding a squeeze of fresh lemon or lime juice to the smoothie bowl base helps prevent any fruit you've mixed into it from browning.

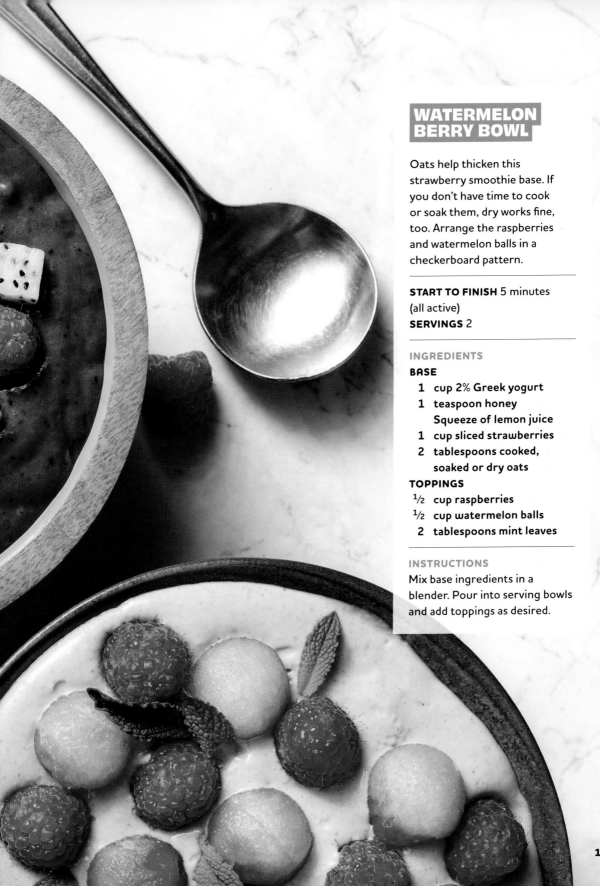

WATERMELON BERRY BOWL

Oats help thicken this strawberry smoothie base. If you don't have time to cook or soak them, dry works fine, too. Arrange the raspberries and watermelon balls in a checkerboard pattern.

START TO FINISH 5 minutes (all active)
SERVINGS 2

INGREDIENTS

BASE
- 1 cup 2% Greek yogurt
- 1 teaspoon honey
  Squeeze of lemon juice
- 1 cup sliced strawberries
- 2 tablespoons cooked, soaked or dry oats

TOPPINGS
- ½ cup raspberries
- ½ cup watermelon balls
- 2 tablespoons mint leaves

INSTRUCTIONS

Mix base ingredients in a blender. Pour into serving bowls and add toppings as desired.

163

CHICKEN BONE BROTH

Bone broth is said to be a potent anti-inflammatory, which aids in brain function, among other benefits. It's also rich in amino acids, which are the body's cellular building blocks. Made in a slow cooker, this broth is flavorful and rich. It will keep in the fridge for five days; freeze for longer storage.

START TO FINISH 15 minutes (plus 1 day inactive)
SERVINGS 24

INGREDIENTS

- 3 **pounds raw chicken bones**
- 1 **large onion, coarsely chopped**
- 1 **tablespoon apple cider vinegar**
- 1 **tablespoon minced garlic**
- 1 **tablespoon sea salt**
- 4 **fresh bay leaves**
- 3 **quarts water**
  GARNISH chopped parsley

INSTRUCTIONS

1 In the pot of a slow cooker, combine bones, onion, vinegar, garlic, salt and bay leaves. Cover with water, stopping at least 1 inch from top of pot.
2 Place lid on slow cooker; cook on low for 24 hours.
3 With a slotted spoon, remove and discard solids.
4 Pour mixture through a strainer; let cool.
5 Transfer to three 1-quart glass jars with lids; store in refrigerator.
6 Garnish with parsley when serving.

TURMERIC CAULIFLOWER SOUP

Curcumin, the active ingredient in the spice turmeric, can help increase the number of connections between neurons.

START TO FINISH 1 hour (5 minutes active)
SERVINGS 4

INGREDIENTS

- 1 (10-ounce) bag cauliflower florets
- 2 shallots, quartered
- 4 cloves garlic, smashed
- 2 tablespoons olive oil
- 1 teaspoon turmeric
- 1 teaspoon cumin
- 1 teaspoon sea salt
- ½ cup red lentils
- 2 cups vegetable broth
- 2½ cups unsweetened cashew milk, divided
- GARNISHES lime wedges, parsley leaves, cracked black pepper, turmeric

INSTRUCTIONS

1 Preheat oven to 425 F.
2 In a large bowl, combine cauliflower, shallots and garlic.
3 Drizzle with olive oil. Add in turmeric, cumin and salt; toss.
4 Spread cauliflower mixture on baking sheet and roast for 30 minutes, stirring halfway through.
5 In a large saucepan, mix roasted cauliflower, lentils, broth and 2 cups cashew milk. Over high heat, bring the mixture to a boil; cover and reduce to a simmer for 20 minutes.
6 Remove from heat; using an immersion blender, blend until smooth. Stir in remaining cashew milk. Serve immediately; garnish as desired.

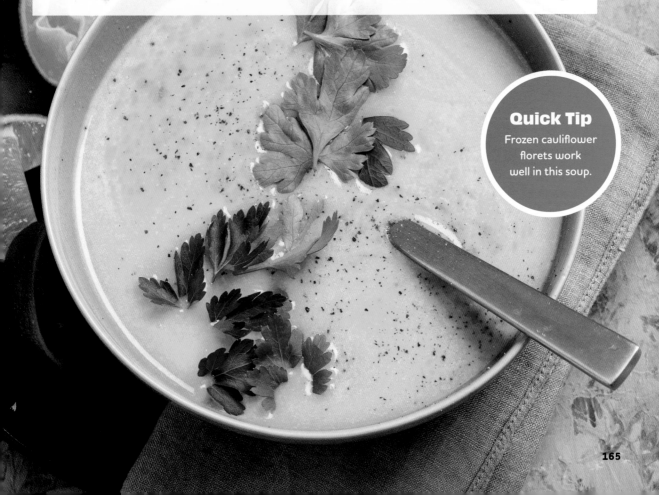

Quick Tip
Frozen cauliflower florets work well in this soup.

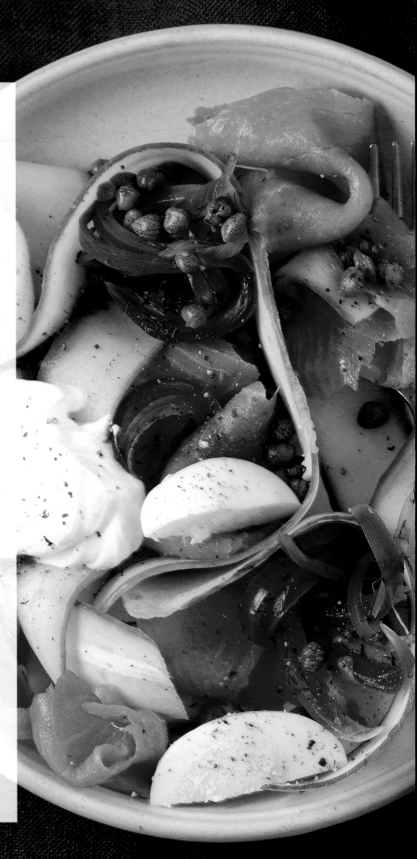

SMOKED SALMON SALAD WITH CUCUMBER RIBBONS AND RED ONION

Pickled onions and gut-healthy yogurt add a nice tartness to this dish, which is high in omega-3s.

START TO FINISH 25 minutes (10 minutes active)
SERVINGS 4

INGREDIENTS

- 1 small red onion, thinly sliced
- 1 cup red wine vinegar
- 1 tablespoon sugar
- 1/2 teaspoon salt
- 1 1/2 teaspoons dried dill
- 1 (8-ounce) package smoked salmon
- 1 English cucumber, skin on, sliced into ribbons
- 2 hard-boiled eggs, quartered
- 1/4 cup Greek yogurt
  GARNISHES cracked black pepper, capers

INSTRUCTIONS

1 In a small saucepan over medium-high heat, add red onion, vinegar, sugar, salt and dill. Bring to a boil. Remove from heat; cover and let stand 15 minutes.

2 Divide among 4 bowls the salmon pieces, cucumber ribbons, eggs and dollops of yogurt. Drain onion mixture and place on top.

3 Top with cracked pepper and capers and serve.

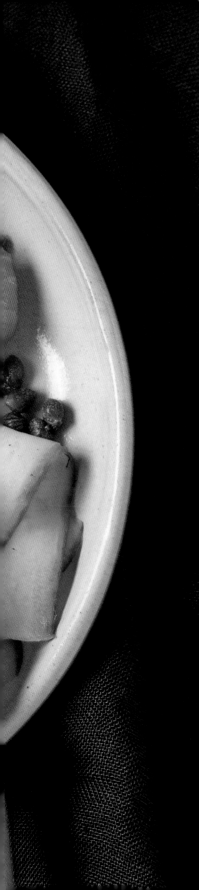

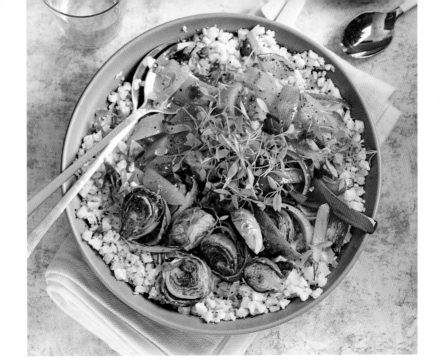

ROASTED VEGETABLE AND CAULIFLOWER RICE BOWL

Enjoy a rainbow of roasted veggies.

START TO FINISH 25 minutes
(10 minutes active)
SERVINGS 2

INGREDIENTS

- 1 orange bell pepper, coarsely chopped
- 1 red onion, sliced
- 1 pound Brussels sprouts, trimmed
- 1 tablespoon plus ¼ cup olive oil, divided
- ½ teaspoon sea salt
- ½ teaspoon ground black pepper
- 2 tablespoons champagne vinegar
- 1 teaspoon Dijon mustard
- 1 (16-ounce) microwavable bag cauliflower rice, cooked according to package directions

GARNISH micro parsley leaves

INSTRUCTIONS

1 Preheat oven to 425 F.
2 On a rimmed sheet pan, add pepper, onion and sprouts.
3 Drizzle with 1 tablespoon olive oil; sprinkle with salt and pepper.
4 Roast for 10 minutes, turning halfway through cooking. Remove from oven.
5 Meanwhile, to make dressing, in a small bowl whisk together ¼ cup olive oil, vinegar and mustard until smooth.
6 Divide the cooked cauliflower rice between 2 individual serving bowls.
7 Top evenly with roasted vegetables; drizzle with dressing.
8 Garnish with micro parsley leaves and serve.

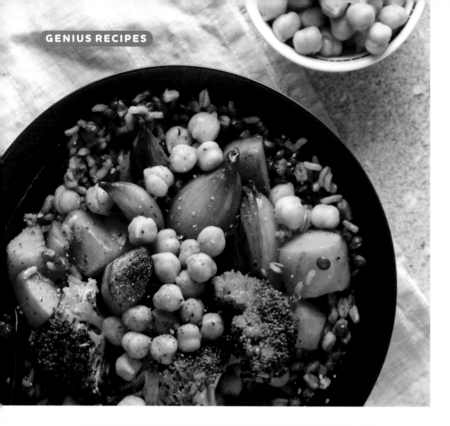

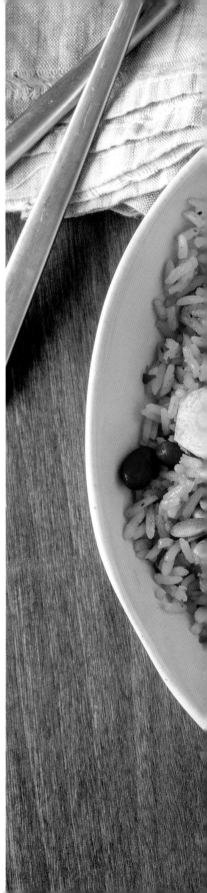

CHICKPEA AND SPELT BOWL WITH ROASTED BROCCOLI AND SHALLOTS

Spelt is an ancient grain. It's a good source of dietary fiber and is rich in iron and phosphorus.

START TO FINISH 25 minutes (10 minutes active)
SERVINGS 2

INGREDIENTS

- 1 cup broccoli florets
- 2 shallots, quartered
- 1 cup cubed butternut squash
- 1 tablespoon avocado or olive oil
- ½ teaspoon sea salt
- ½ teaspoon ground black pepper
- 1 (8-ounce) package microwavable spelt, green lentils and long-grain brown rice, cooked according to package directions
- 1 (15.5-ounce) can chickpeas, drained and rinsed

INSTRUCTIONS

1 Preheat oven to 400 F.
2 On a rimmed sheet pan, place broccoli florets, shallots and squash. Drizzle with oil; sprinkle with salt and pepper.
3 Roast in oven for 10 minutes or until vegetables are browned, turning halfway through cooking. Remove from oven.
4 Divide the spelt, green lentils and brown rice mix between 2 individual serving bowls.
5 Top each bowl with roasted vegetables and chickpeas.

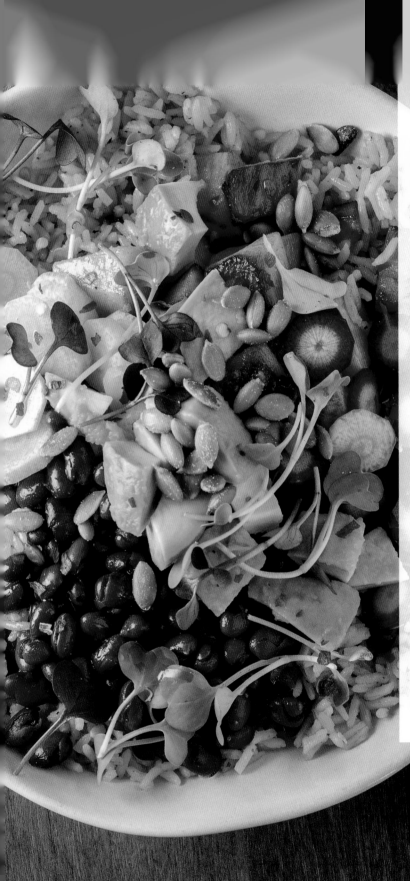

POWER BOWL

Butternut squash is full of
vitamins, minerals and fiber.
Carrots add color and crunch,
as well as beta-carotene, which
may help keep the brain younger.

START TO FINISH 15 minutes
(all active)
SERVINGS 2

INGREDIENTS

1 (8-ounce) microwavable
   bag turmeric rice, cooked
   according to package
   directions
1 (15-ounce) can black
   beans, drained and rinsed
1 cup cubed and cooked
   butternut squash
1 small yellow carrot, sliced
1 small purple carrot, sliced
1 small avocado, coarsely
   chopped
¼ cup roasted pepitas
¼ teaspoon red pepper flakes
   GARNISH radish
   microgreens

INSTRUCTIONS

1 Divide the cooked turmeric
rice between 2 individual
serving bowls.
2 Evenly top with black beans,
squash, carrots, avocado,
pepitas and red pepper flakes.
3 Garnish with radish
microgreens to serve.

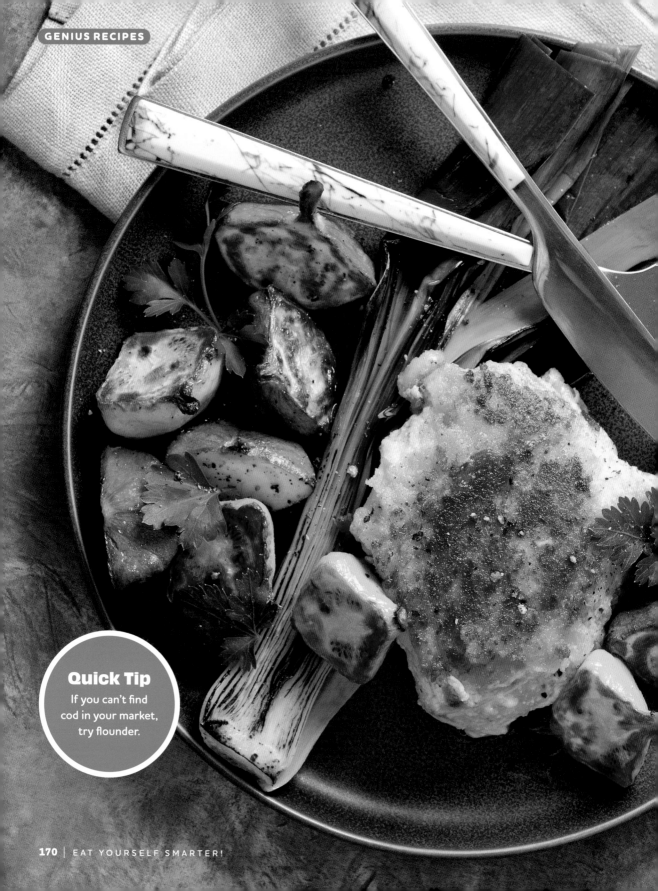

Quick Tip

If you can't find cod in your market, try flounder.

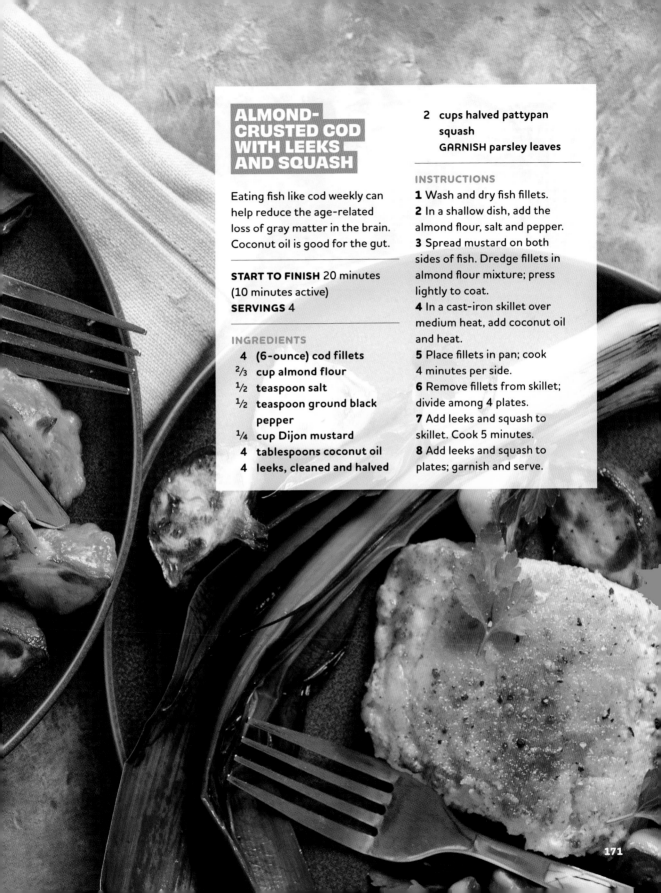

ALMOND-CRUSTED COD WITH LEEKS AND SQUASH

Eating fish like cod weekly can help reduce the age-related loss of gray matter in the brain. Coconut oil is good for the gut.

START TO FINISH 20 minutes (10 minutes active)
SERVINGS 4

INGREDIENTS

- 4 (6-ounce) cod fillets
- ²/₃ cup almond flour
- ½ teaspoon salt
- ½ teaspoon ground black pepper
- ¼ cup Dijon mustard
- 4 tablespoons coconut oil
- 4 leeks, cleaned and halved
- 2 cups halved pattypan squash
- GARNISH parsley leaves

INSTRUCTIONS

1 Wash and dry fish fillets.
2 In a shallow dish, add the almond flour, salt and pepper.
3 Spread mustard on both sides of fish. Dredge fillets in almond flour mixture; press lightly to coat.
4 In a cast-iron skillet over medium heat, add coconut oil and heat.
5 Place fillets in pan; cook 4 minutes per side.
6 Remove fillets from skillet; divide among 4 plates.
7 Add leeks and squash to skillet. Cook 5 minutes.
8 Add leeks and squash to plates; garnish and serve.

HERB-CRUSTED SALMON FILLETS WITH TOMATO AND OREGANO SALAD

Herbs give the salmon in this healthy-fat-filled recipe a Greek flair. Serve with lemon wedges; the citrus and fish pair perfectly.

START TO FINISH 20 minutes (5 minutes active)
SERVINGS 4

INGREDIENTS

- 4 (6-ounce) salmon fillets
- ½ teaspoon salt
- ½ teaspoon ground black pepper
- 1 tablespoon chopped chives
- 1 tablespoon dill
- 1 tablespoon thyme
- 2 tablespoons avocado oil
- 1 pint cherry tomatoes, halved
- ¼ cup olive oil
- 2 cups mixed salad greens
  GARNISHES oregano leaves, dill sprigs

INSTRUCTIONS

1 Sprinkle salmon fillets with salt, pepper and herbs.
2 In a cast-iron skillet over medium-high heat, heat avocado oil.
3 Add fillets to pan. Cook 3 minutes per side or until cooked through.
4 In a large bowl, toss tomatoes with olive oil.
5 Divide salad greens among 4 dinner plates.
6 Top salad with salmon and tomatoes. Garnish and serve.

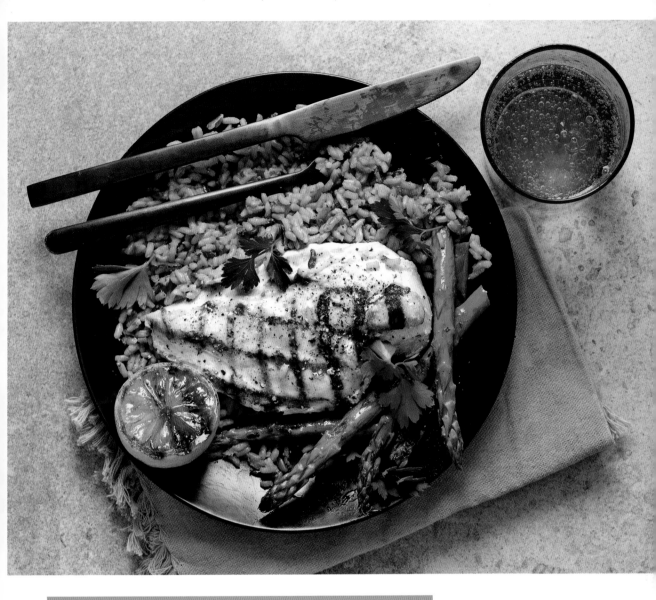

GRILLED LEMON CHICKEN AND ASPARAGUS

Add other veggies, such as baby spinach, to boost the brain-health benefits. Serve with a side of brown rice or other whole grain.

START TO FINISH 20 minutes (10 minutes active)
SERVINGS 4

INGREDIENTS

- 4 **boneless, skinless chicken breasts**
- ½ **teaspoon salt**
- ½ **teaspoon ground black pepper**
- 1 **tablespoon avocado oil**
- 1 **pound asparagus, trimmed**
- 2 **lemons, halved**
  GARNISH parsley leaves

INSTRUCTIONS

1 Sprinkle both sides of chicken breasts with salt and pepper.

2 Brush a grill pan with oil; place pan over medium-high heat.

3 Place chicken in grill pan; cook 3 to 4 minutes per side or until done.

4 Set chicken aside; keep warm. In the same pan, place asparagus and lemon halves; cook for 2 minutes.

5 Divide chicken, asparagus and lemon halves among 4 dinner plates; garnish with parsley.

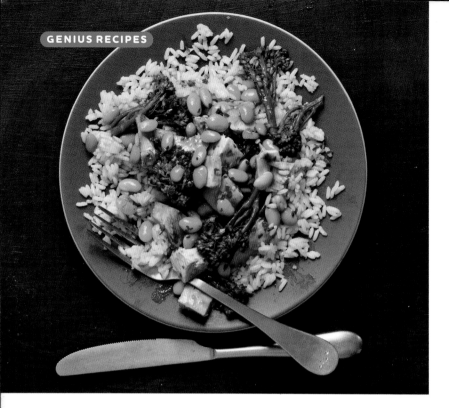

SESAME GARLIC CHICKEN WITH BROCCOLI RABE

Broccoli rabe adds a nutty, earthy, slightly bitter taste (and great brain-health benefits) to this dish. Parcook it by boiling it for 1 minute in salted water, then plunging it into ice water.

START TO FINISH 15 minutes
(5 minutes active)
SERVINGS 4

INGREDIENTS

- 1 tablespoon sesame oil
- 1 tablespoon chili oil
- 4 boneless, skinless chicken breasts, cubed
- ½ teaspoon salt
- ¼ teaspoon ground black pepper
- 1 (8.8-ounce) package precooked rice, microwaved according to package directions
- ½ pound broccoli rabe, parcooked then lightly sauteed or steamed as desired until warm
- ¼ cup cooked edamame (frozen or fresh)
- 1 (12-ounce) bottle garlic-chili sauce
  GARNISH red pepper flakes

INSTRUCTIONS

1 In a skillet over medium-high heat, add sesame and chili oils.
2 Sprinkle chicken evenly with salt and pepper. Add chicken to skillet; cook, stirring constantly, for 6 minutes.
3 Meanwhile, divide warm rice evenly among 4 individual plates. Top with cooked chicken, broccoli rabe and edamame.
4 Drizzle with garlic-chili sauce and garnish to serve.

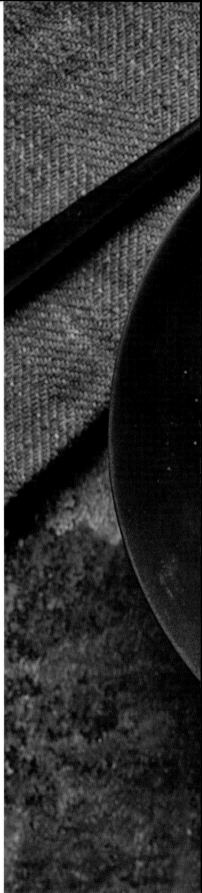

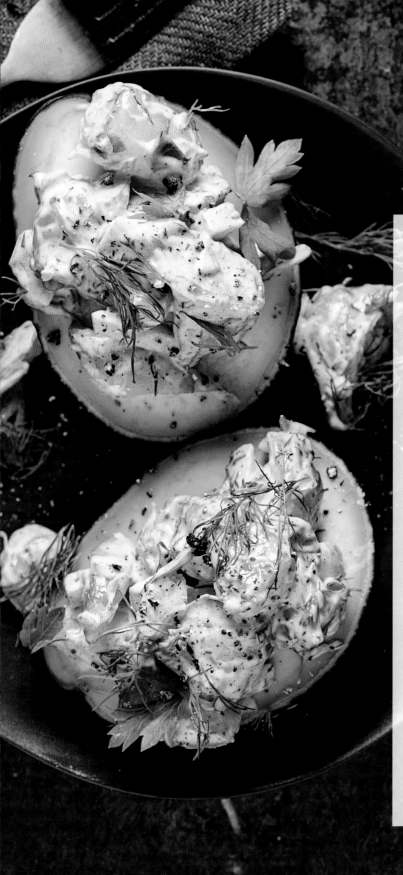

SHRIMP SALAD-STUFFED AVOCADOS

Cut a small slice off the base of each avocado half so it sits upright on the serving plate.

START TO FINISH 15 minutes (10 minutes active)
SERVINGS 2

INGREDIENTS

¼ cup mayonnaise
3 tablespoons chopped celery
3 tablespoons sliced scallions
2 teaspoons chopped parsley
1 teaspoon chopped dill
1 tablespoon lemon juice
1 tablespoon Old Bay seasoning
½ pound cooked shrimp, roughly chopped
2 ripe avocados, halved and pitted (do not peel)
GARNISHES dill sprigs, chopped parsley

INSTRUCTIONS

1 In a medium bowl, combine mayonnaise and next 7 ingredients. Stir well to mix.
2 Fill the avocado halves with the shrimp salad mixture and garnish to serve.

ASPARAGUS SALAD WITH PISTACHIOS

Asparagus may help reduce the blues and prevent irritability.

START TO FINISH 15 minutes (all active)
SERVINGS 4

INGREDIENTS

- ½ cup toasted pistachios
- 2 pounds raw asparagus, trimmed and sliced
- 1 teaspoon lemon zest
- 1 tablespoon lemon juice
- 1 teaspoon salt
- ⅛ teaspoon red pepper flakes
- ⅓ cup extra-virgin olive oil
- ½ cup shaved Parmesan cheese
- GARNISH mint leaves

INSTRUCTIONS

1 In a serving bowl, toss pistachios and asparagus.
2 To make dressing, in a small bowl, whisk together lemon zest, lemon juice, salt, red pepper flakes, olive oil and Parmesan cheese.
3 Pour dressing over pistachios and asparagus; toss and garnish to serve.

Quick Tip

If you've never had raw asparagus, this is a perfect way to try it. Cut stalks on the diagonal into thin slices; this way, they're more tender and soak up more flavor from the seasonings, too.

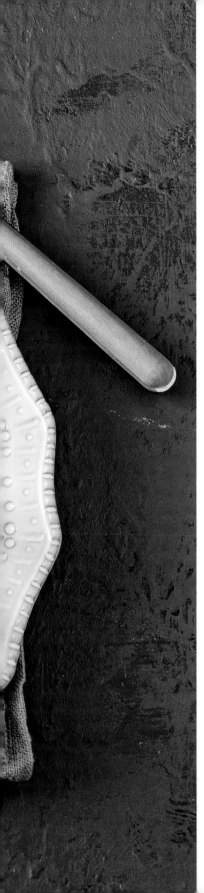

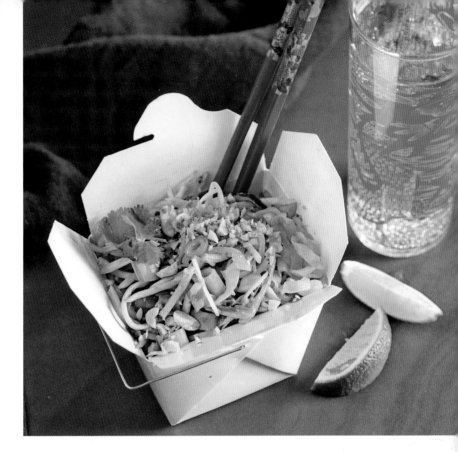

PAD THAI NOODLES

This classic dish gets a low-carb makeover. Toss in any antioxidant-rich veggies you like.

START TO FINISH 10 minutes (all active)
SERVINGS 4

INGREDIENTS

- 1 (12-ounce) bag broccoli slaw mix
- ¼ cup sliced scallions
- 4 cups shirataki noodles, drained and rinsed (we used Skinny Pasta konjac fettuccine)
- ¼ cup chopped dry-roasted peanuts
- ½ cup sugar-free peanut butter
- 2 tablespoons sesame oil
- 2 tablespoons lime juice
- 2 tablespoons water
- 1 teaspoon chopped ginger
- 1 teaspoon chopped garlic
- ½ teaspoon salt
  GARNISHES cilantro sprigs, lime wedges

INSTRUCTIONS

1 In a large bowl, combine slaw mix, scallions, noodles and peanuts.
2 In a blender, add peanut butter and remaining ingredients; blend until smooth.
3 Pour dressing over slaw mixture; toss gently.
4 Garnish to serve.

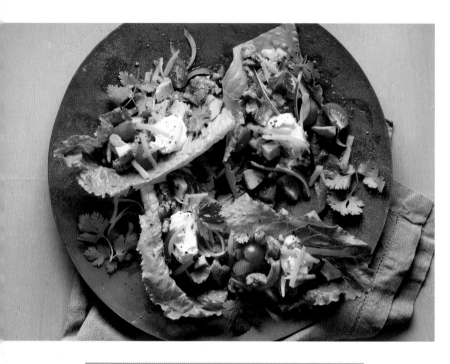

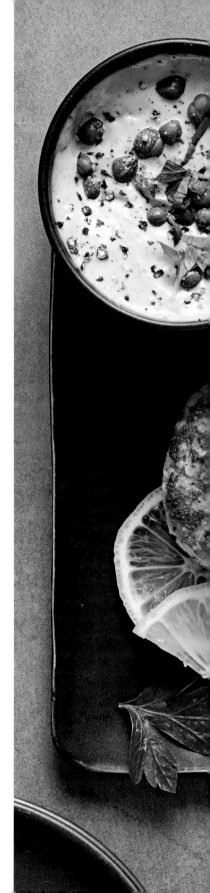

TURKEY TACO LETTUCE WRAPS

This low-carb meal helps keep your brain nourished without making you feel sluggish.

START TO FINISH 20 minutes (12 minutes active)
SERVINGS 4

INGREDIENTS

  2 **tablespoons olive oil**
 ½ **cup chopped onion**
  1 **pound ground turkey**
  1 **teaspoon minced garlic**
 ½ **teaspoon salt**
 ½ **teaspoon ground black pepper**
  1 **tablespoon chili powder**
  1 **teaspoon cumin**
 ¼ **cup tomato sauce**
 ¼ **cup chicken stock**
  8 **romaine lettuce leaves**

GARNISHES shredded cheddar cheese, quartered cherry tomatoes, diced avocado, sliced red onion, sour cream, cilantro sprigs

INSTRUCTIONS

1 In a large skillet over medium-high heat, heat olive oil. Add onion; saute for 2 minutes. Add turkey and garlic; cook 5 to 6 minutes or until no longer pink. Season with salt and pepper.
2 Add chili powder, cumin, tomato sauce and stock to skillet. Lower heat; simmer 5 minutes or until thickened.
3 Place lettuce leaves on plates; top with mixture and serve garnishes on the side.

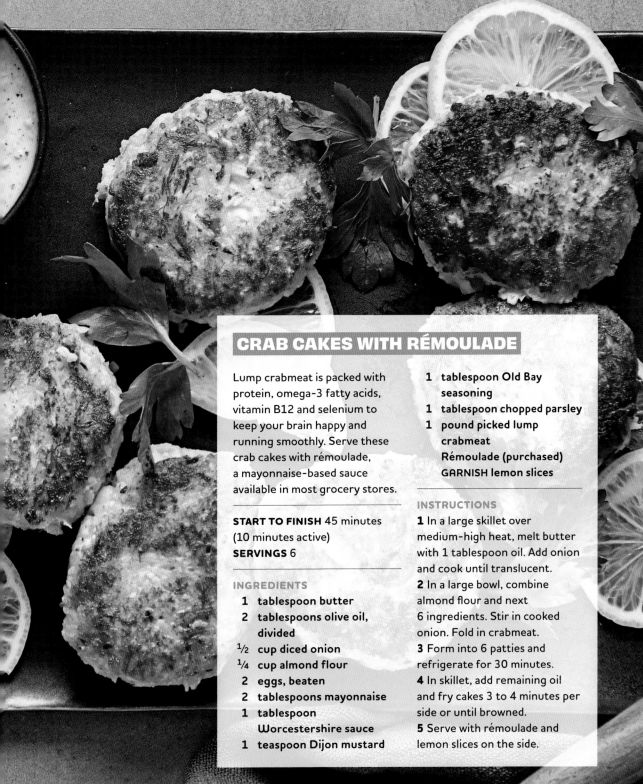

CRAB CAKES WITH RÉMOULADE

Lump crabmeat is packed with protein, omega-3 fatty acids, vitamin B12 and selenium to keep your brain happy and running smoothly. Serve these crab cakes with rémoulade, a mayonnaise-based sauce available in most grocery stores.

START TO FINISH 45 minutes (10 minutes active)
SERVINGS 6

INGREDIENTS

- 1 tablespoon butter
- 2 tablespoons olive oil, divided
- ½ cup diced onion
- ¼ cup almond flour
- 2 eggs, beaten
- 2 tablespoons mayonnaise
- 1 tablespoon Worcestershire sauce
- 1 teaspoon Dijon mustard
- 1 tablespoon Old Bay seasoning
- 1 tablespoon chopped parsley
- 1 pound picked lump crabmeat
- Rémoulade (purchased)
- GARNISH lemon slices

INSTRUCTIONS

1 In a large skillet over medium-high heat, melt butter with 1 tablespoon oil. Add onion and cook until translucent.
2 In a large bowl, combine almond flour and next 6 ingredients. Stir in cooked onion. Fold in crabmeat.
3 Form into 6 patties and refrigerate for 30 minutes.
4 In skillet, add remaining oil and fry cakes 3 to 4 minutes per side or until browned.
5 Serve with rémoulade and lemon slices on the side.

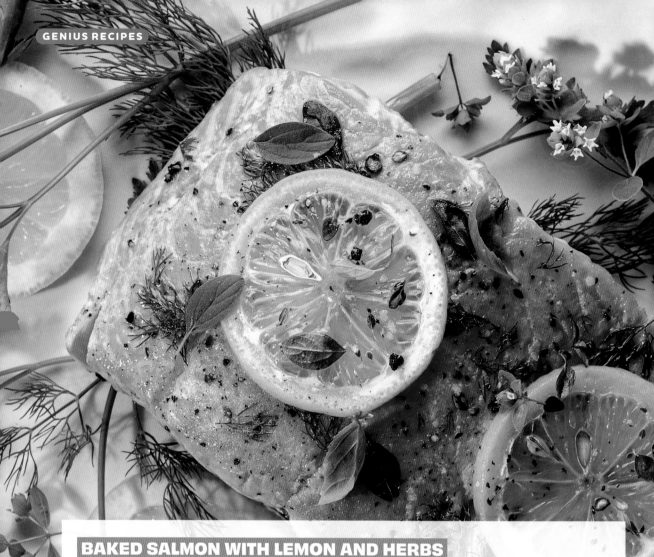

BAKED SALMON WITH LEMON AND HERBS

Salmon is one of the healthiest fish and pairs well with a variety of seasonings. This version is super easy to make on a busy night.

START TO FINISH 20 minutes (5 minutes active)
SERVINGS 4

INGREDIENTS

- ¼ cup butter, divided
- 1 teaspoon minced garlic
- 2 tablespoons chopped parsley
- ½ teaspoon sea salt
- ¼ teaspoon ground black pepper
- 2 pounds salmon fillets, cut into 4 portions
- 1 large lemon, sliced
  GARNISHES lemon slices, basil leaves, parsley sprigs, thyme sprigs, oregano sprigs

INSTRUCTIONS

1 Preheat oven to 400 F.
2 Place 2 tablespoons butter on a rimmed baking sheet. Place in oven to melt.
3 In a small pan, melt the remaining butter; whisk in garlic, parsley, salt and pepper.
4 Remove baking pan from oven; place salmon fillets, skin-side down, on pan. Arrange lemon slices on fillets and pour garlic butter over top.
5 Roast for 10 to 12 minutes, until the fish is cooked to desired doneness.
6 Transfer to a serving platter; spoon garlic butter from pan onto fillets and garnish to serve.

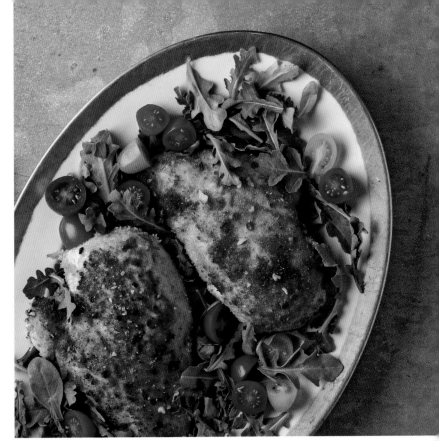
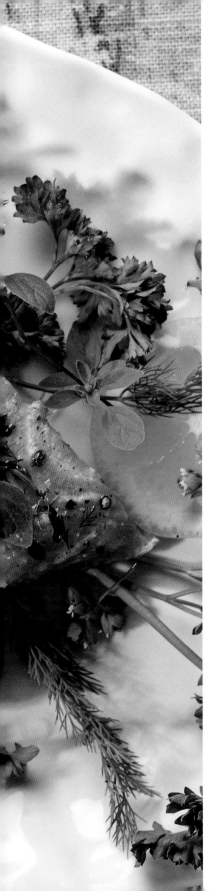

PISTACHIO-CRUSTED CHICKEN BREASTS

Pistachios provide a tasty crunch and healthy fats to this dish. Press the crust firmly to the chicken to make sure the nuts adhere well.

START TO FINISH 45 minutes (10 minutes active)
SERVINGS 2

INGREDIENTS
- ½ cup pistachios
- ½ cup almond flour
- 2 boneless, skinless chicken breasts, about 1½ inches thick
- 2 tablespoons mustard
  GARNISHES arugula, cherry tomatoes

INSTRUCTIONS
1 Preheat oven to 400 F.
2 In a food processor, pulse the pistachios until they have the texture of breadcrumbs.
3 In a shallow dish, combine pistachios and almond flour.
4 Brush both sides of each chicken breast with mustard. Dip chicken into pistachio mixture, pressing firmly to adhere.
5 Coat a baking sheet with vegetable oil cooking spray. Arrange chicken on sheet so pieces are not touching. Bake 25 to 35 minutes or until cooked through.
6 Transfer to serving platter; garnish to serve.

BROWN RICE ALMOND MILK PUDDING

Brown rice gives this dessert a delicious nutty taste, and it's higher in protein, antioxidants and fiber than white rice.

START TO FINISH 1 hour 5 minutes (5 minutes active)
SERVINGS 4

INGREDIENTS

- 1 cup brown rice
- 4 cups unsweetened almond milk, divided
- 1 tablespoon maple syrup
- 2 teaspoons vanilla
- 1/4 teaspoon ground nutmeg
- 1/8 teaspoon ground cinnamon
- 1/8 teaspoon salt
- 1/4 cup golden raisins
  GARNISH ground cinnamon

INSTRUCTIONS

1 In a small Dutch oven, add brown rice, 3 cups almond milk, maple syrup, vanilla, nutmeg, cinnamon and salt.

2 Bring to a boil over medium-high heat.

3 Reduce heat to low, cover and simmer for 45 minutes, stirring occasionally.

4 Add remaining 1 cup almond milk; let simmer an additional 15 minutes or until rice is soft and chewy.

5 Stir in raisins and garnish to serve.

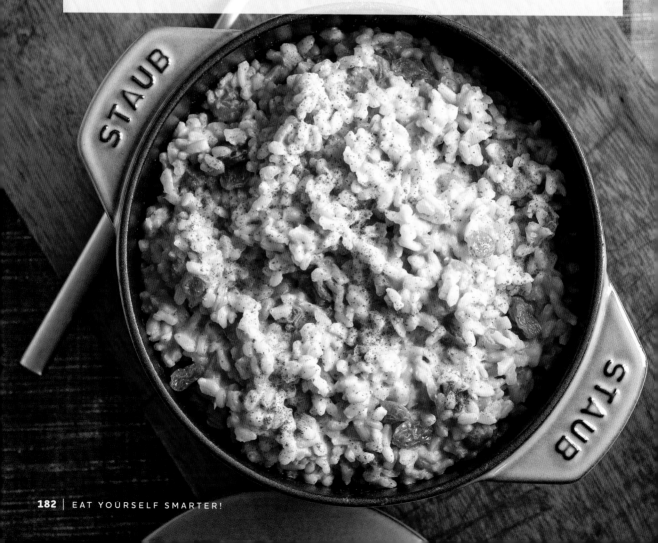

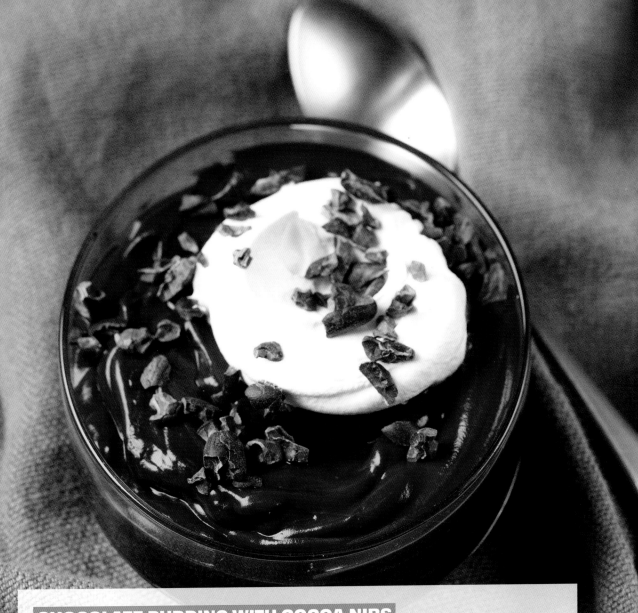

CHOCOLATE PUDDING WITH COCOA NIBS

This is a super-healthy dessert or snack option, thanks to chia seeds, protein powder and dark cocoa. Cocoa and cacao nibs are naturally low in sugar, and maple syrup won't cause blood sugar to spike, so it's a smart indulgence.

START TO FINISH 65 minutes (5 minutes active)

SERVINGS 4

INGREDIENTS

  2 cups unsweetened almond milk
  6 tablespoons chia seeds
  ½ cup vegan chocolate protein powder
  ¼ cup dark cocoa powder
  ¼ cup maple syrup

GARNISHES whipped coconut cream, cocoa nibs

INSTRUCTIONS

1 In a blender, mix all ingredients on high for 30 seconds.
2 Pour into 4 serving bowls; chill in refrigerator for 1 hour. Garnish to serve.

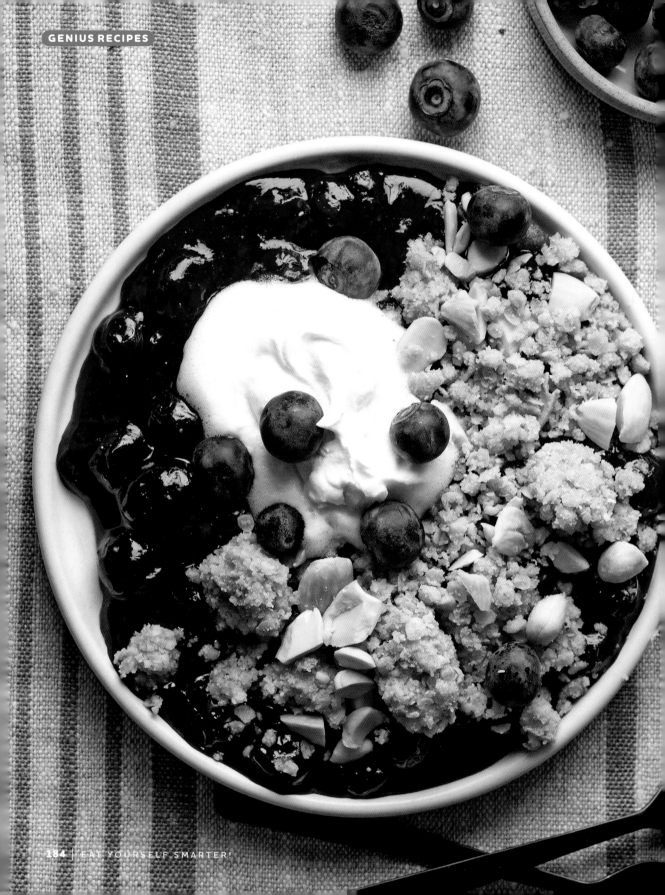

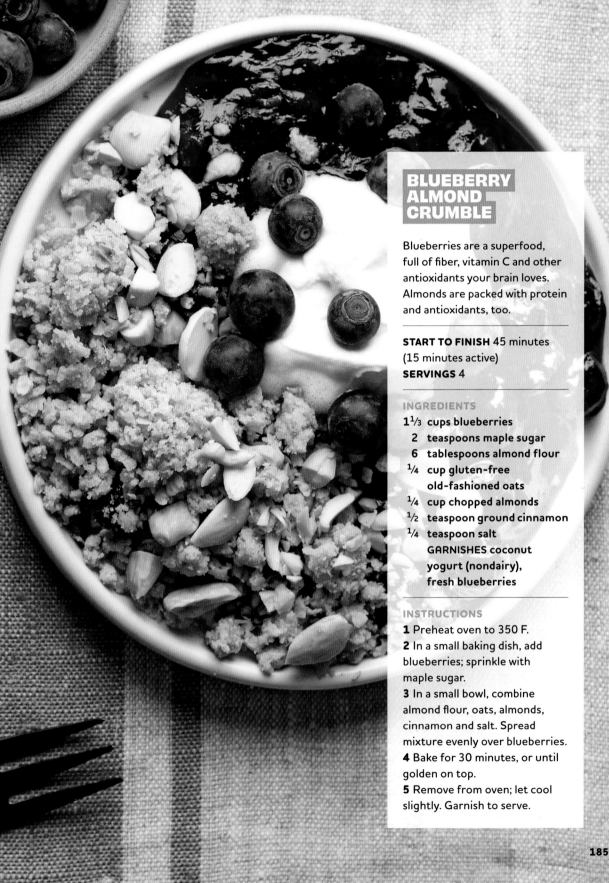

BLUEBERRY ALMOND CRUMBLE

Blueberries are a superfood, full of fiber, vitamin C and other antioxidants your brain loves. Almonds are packed with protein and antioxidants, too.

START TO FINISH 45 minutes (15 minutes active)
SERVINGS 4

INGREDIENTS

1⅓ cups blueberries
2 teaspoons maple sugar
6 tablespoons almond flour
¼ cup gluten-free old-fashioned oats
¼ cup chopped almonds
½ teaspoon ground cinnamon
¼ teaspoon salt
GARNISHES coconut yogurt (nondairy), fresh blueberries

INSTRUCTIONS

1 Preheat oven to 350 F.
2 In a small baking dish, add blueberries; sprinkle with maple sugar.
3 In a small bowl, combine almond flour, oats, almonds, cinnamon and salt. Spread mixture evenly over blueberries.
4 Bake for 30 minutes, or until golden on top.
5 Remove from oven; let cool slightly. Garnish to serve.

SPECIAL THANKS TO CONTRIBUTING WRITERS

Sherry Baker ✳ Barbara Brody ✳ Claire Connors ✳ Carlin Flora ✳ Kimberly Goad
Phillip Rhodes ✳ Deborah Skolnik

CREDITS

DISCLAIMER

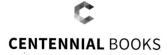

CENTENNIAL BOOKS

An Imprint of
Centennial Media, LLC
1111 Brickell Avenue, 10th Floor
Miami, FL 33131, U.S.A.

ISBN 978-1-951274-93-1

Distributed by
Simon & Schuster, Inc.
1230 Avenue of the Americas
New York, NY 10020, U.S.A.

For information about custom editions, special sales and premium and corporate purchases,
please contact Centennial Media at contact@centennialmedia.com.

Manufactured in China

10 9 8 7 6 5 4 3 2 1

PUBLISHERS & CO-FOUNDERS Ben Harris, Sebastian Raatz
EDITORIAL DIRECTOR Annabel Vered
CREATIVE DIRECTOR Jessica Power
EXECUTIVE EDITOR Janet Giovanelli
FEATURES EDITOR Alyssa Shaffer
DEPUTY EDITORS Ron Kelly, Anne Marie O'Connor
MANAGING EDITOR Lisa Chambers
DESIGN DIRECTOR Martin Elfers
SENIOR ART DIRECTOR Pino Impastato
ART DIRECTORS Runyon Hall, Jaclyn Loney, Natali Suasnavas, Joseph Ulatowski
COPY/PRODUCTION Patty Carroll, Angela Taormina
SENIOR PHOTO EDITOR Jenny Veiga
PHOTO EDITOR Keri Pruett
PRODUCTION MANAGER Paul Rodina
PRODUCTION ASSISTANT Alyssa Swiderski
EDITORIAL ASSISTANT Tiana Schippa
SALES & MARKETING Jeremy Nurnberg